Race in Contemporary Medicine

With the first patent being granted to "BiDil," a combined medication that is deemed to be most effective for a specific "race," African-Americans for a specific form of heart failure, the on-going debate about the effect of the older category of race has been renewed. What role should "race" in the discussion of genetic alleles and populations today?

The new genetics has seemed to make "race" both a category that is seen useful if not necessary. Should one think about "race" as a transitional category that is of some use while we continue to explore the actual genetic makeup and relationships in populations? Or is such a transitional solution poisoning the actual research and practice?

Race in Contemporary Medicine will focus on these questions from a bio-medical and social perspective and discusses issues such as:

- Does "race" present both epidemiological and a historical problem for the society in which it is raised as well as for medical research and practice?
- Who defines "race" – the self-defined group, the government, the research funder, the researcher?
- What does one do with what are deemed "race" specific diseases such as "Jewish genetic diseases" that are so defined because they are often concentrated in a group but are also found beyond the group?
- Are we comfortable designating "Jews" or "African-Americans" as "races" given their genetic diversity? The book will focus on these questions from a bio-medical and social perspective.

This book was previously published as a special issue of *Patterns of Prejudice*.

Sander L. Gilman is distinguished professor of the Liberal Arts and Sciences at Emory University.

Race in Contemporary Medicine

Edited by
Sander L. Gilman

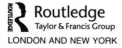
Routledge
Taylor & Francis Group

LONDON AND NEW YORK

First published 2008 by Routledge
2 Park Square, Milton Park, Abingdon, Oxon, OX14 4RN

Simultaneously published in the USA and Canada
by Routledge
270 Madison Avenue, New York, NY 10016

Routledge is an imprint of the Taylor & Francis Group, an informa business

Typeset in Palatino by Datapage International Ltd, Dublin, Ireland
Printed and bound in Great Britain by MPG Books Ltd, Bodmin, Cornwall

British Library Cataloguing in Publication Data
A catalogue record for this book is available from the British Library

ISBN 10: 0-415-41365-6 hbk
ISBN 13: 978-0-415-41365-7 hbk

Contents

Introduction: race and contemporary medicine
Sander L. Gilman   vii

1. Blood and stories: how genomics is rewriting race, medicine
   and human history
   Priscilla Wald   1

2. Alcohol and the Jews (again), race and medicine (again):
   on race and medicine in historical perspective
   Sander L. Gilman   32

3. Reflections on race and the biologization of difference
   Katya Gibel Azoulay   50

4. Folk taxonomy, prejudice and the human genome: using
   disease as a Jewish ethnic marker
   Judith S. Neulander   77

5. Eugenics and the racial genome: politics at the molecular
   level
   Sharon L. Snyder and David T. Mitchell   95

6. The risky gene: epidemiology and the evolution of race
   Philip Alcabes   109

7. The molecular reinscription of race: unanticipated issues in
   biotechnology and forensic science
   Troy Duster   122

8. Biobanks of a 'racial kind': mining for difference in the new
   genetics
   Sandra Soo-Jin Lee   137

9. The rhetoric of race in breast cancer research
   Kelly E. Happe   155

10. Against racial medicine
    Joseph L. Graves, Jr and Michael R. Rose   175

Index   189

Introduction: race and contemporary medicine

*R*ace and Contemporary Medicine is concerned with the reappearance of 'race' as a category of scientific analysis within the world of medicine. But it also reflects on the cultural implications of race from the nineteenth to the twenty-first centuries. For medical culture is also part of general culture; and general culture has been shaped at least since the Enlightenment by the findings and claims of the 'hottest' areas of the 'new' medicine. The 'two cultures' are actually one: each mirroring and distorting the other; each having its own assumed audience yet encompassing, for good or ill, all audiences.

There was a conscious attempt in the early twentieth century to transform 'race' into 'ethnicity' and yet biological explanations continued to define all realms of human difference. The movement from biological to cultural explanations for human activity a century ago was not smooth. In all cases cross-contamination of models of explanation and analysis took place. After the Holocaust, after the racial politics of extermination in the Third Reich, after the American civil rights movement, racial explanations for pathologies were given less and less credence, at least in public. 'Race' seemed to be a category unlikely to be repatriated from the exile of 'bad' science and 'quack' medicine. Who after the Nuremburg doctors' trial would have dared to use 'race' as a category of analysis without risking public opprobrium?

The radical changes in the meaning of 'race' at the end of the twentieth century (and its transvaluation within self-defined 'racial' communities) saw a rethinking of the notion. Today we are again grappling with an attempt to 'lump' human beings into biologically defined populations. We are doing so with the aid of a new and often exciting science, namely, human genetics. The proliferation of genetic explanations for 'disease', from breast cancer to addiction, has called forth critical voices. Yet we are also convinced of the possibility of a genetic determinant for many diseases, following the model of clearly defined, inherited pathologies, such as Huntington's chorea. They provide a means by which medicine imagines the genetics of disease as clearly interpretable and demonstrable. What happens when a biological definition of identity becomes a compelling aspect of community self-definition? What happens when the 'Jews' or 'African Americans' or 'Asians' begin to think of themselves as a virtual family interconnected by their biological inheritance? And what happens when the markers for such affiliation are shared diseases?

In February 2005, for Black History Month, Henry Louis Gates, Jr, who had edited one of the most important books on these subjects, *'Race,' Writing and Difference* (1986), presented a four-hour public television show entitled *African-American Lives*. Profiled were a series of African-American celebrities from Oprah Winfrey to Gates himself. The first two-hour programme used traditional genealogical tools to trace the ancestry of subjects back into the world of American slavery. The second, much more contentious programme used the tools of DNA research to pinpoint their genealogy before the Middle Passage. The forensic DNA research was based on the assumption that what was to be identified was the subjects' African roots, and it made use of a huge database compiled by Rick Kittles at Ohio State University, which contains over 20,000 lineages from more than 389 indigenous African populations. The shock of the results was that Gates's subjects showed 'Native American' or 'European' ancestry in addition to their 'African' ancestry. Indeed, Gates ironically commented that, as he was only 50 per cent 'African', he might be forced to give up the chair of the Department of African and African-American Studies at Harvard University. Of course, these categories ('African', 'European' or 'Native American') say little about culture or location. Indeed, they say little even about genetic make-up. Popular culture sees genetics as a new form of alchemy, revealing the 'essence' of a person, and uses that essence to define difference, for good or for ill.

It is intriguing that a similar fascination with biology and identity was apparent when, during December 2005, the first face transplant took place in France, reconstructing the mangled face of Isabelle Dinoire. Would her new face give her a new identity? Much concern was expressed about the uniqueness of the face.

> In some ineffable way, though, a person's face *is* the person, inseparable from her external identity and her sense of self. As Ralph Waldo Emerson wrote: 'A man finds room in the few square inches of the face for the traits of all his ancestors; for the expression of all his history, and his wants.'[1]

The sense was that the face transplant was not 'merely' cosmetic.

> The face has always been central to a person's identity. It's how we think of each other, how we reflect emotion and pain, and its primacy is reflected in our language. We 'face the music' or 'put our best face forward.' When your reputation is damaged, you have 'lost face.' In other words, how you look is not simply a matter of vanity.[2]

Our face, like our genes, functions as a public sign of our uniqueness as we more and more fear the complexity of what it means to be unique.

1 'Behind the mask: face transplant reveals mystery of identity', *Dallas Morning News*, 8 December 2005, editorial page.
2 Stephen Kiehl, 'Her new face gives woman a "normal life"', *Baltimore Sun*, 7 February 2006, 1C.

The popular power of the new genetics, as Dorothy Nelkin and Susan Lindee have shown in detail, is only part of the story.[3] One could argue that this is merely a misapprehension or maladaptation of a clear and well-reasoned science. Yet there are compelling scientific reasons why we must concern ourselves with not only nomenclature but also the rationales of science. 'Race' is a label: but it also provides a set of cultural presuppositions about the nature of human beings. Francis Collins, head of the American Human Genome Project, recently commented: 'The downside of using race, whether in research or in the practice of medicine', he says,

> is that we are reifying it as if it has more biological significance than it deserves. Race is an imperfect surrogate for the causative information we seek. To the extent that we continue to use it, we are suggesting to the rest of the world that it is very reliable and that racial categories have more biological meaning than they do. We may even appear to suggest something that I know is not true: that there are bright lines between populations and that races are biologically distinct.[4]

The desire to draw these 'bright lines' is perhaps intrinsic to human nature. The need to define and control, to identify the source of succour or fear, is built into all social groups as central to their self-definition. We know what we are and what we are not. Indeed, part of the fear created by the new genetics is that we may be revealed to be quite different than we imagined ourselves to be. We may be 'ill' (or at risk of transmitting that illness to our offspring) or we may belong to a quite different social group than those with whom we have identified. The power of science is that it seems to 'tell truths'. These truths, as we have known since at least the 1930s, are always framed by the implications of science in the general culture in which it finds itself and which it, in turn, shapes. This does not vitiate the claims of science but urges us constantly to ask about the 'bright lines' it draws.

Thus, *Race and Contemporary Medicine* is a report on a set of questions in transition. It is state of the art as of now: what we do know is that, as the rethinking of the meaning of genetics shifts, as we learn more and more about the complexity of the genome and the even greater complexity of how our genetic make-up interacts with our multilayered experience of the world, all of these debates will also change. The present volume is thus an attempt to deal with the 'bright lines' as they are now constituted. The various contributions approach this from radically different perspectives.

---

3 Dorothy Nelkin and M. Susan Lindee, *The DNA Mystique: The Gene as Cultural Icon* (New York: W. H. Freeman & Co. 1995).

4 Quoted in 'Race and medicine: not a black and white question', *The Economist*, 12 April 2006, 80. This view has recently been put in Keith Wailoo and Stephen Pemberton, *The Troubled Dream of Genetic Medicine: Ethnicity and Innovation in Tay-Sachs, Cystic Fibrosis, and Sickle Cell Disease* (Baltimore, MD: Johns Hopkins University Press 2006).

Priscilla Wald begins the volume looking at the narratives about biological relationships in the newest genomic literature. The biologization of the past is also the theme of my essay on the trajectory of the argument that Jews have a 'natural' resistance to alcoholism, which has now become a commonplace in the contemporary genetics of behaviour. Katya Gibel Azoulay, one of the most astute commentators on the history of race in the United States, shows how the complexity of race is part of a narrative of general culture in which scientific culture is embedded and which scientific culture also helps shape.

As 'race' in the United States tends to be a code term for White–Black difference, the fact that other definable groups, such as the Jews, were (and are again) considered as biological subgroups is the theme of Judith S. Neulander's study of folk taxonomy and 'Jewish genetic diseases'. While the disabled were never considered a race, they were almost always lumped with racial groups in speaking about the negative aspects of human diversity. Sharon L. Snyder and David T. Mitchell examine the parallels and differences in their insightful examination of the politics of eugenics and the racial genome.

Philip Alcabes turns to the question of models of public health and the explosion of concern with 'risk' that comes along with the renewed interest in biological explanations for disease. Troy Duster, the sociologist who has shaped much of the discussion about the reappearance in the biological sciences of arguments about racial difference since the early 1990s, looks at the recent claims of biotechnology and its unforeseen social implications, particularly with regard to forensic science. Sandra Soo-Jin Lee looks at the 'biobank', the DNA repository, as both a physical and symbolic space for notions of genetic essence among human groups in which, despite ubiquitous rhetorical statements to the contrary, race is naturalized. Breast cancer has, at least for the past decade, been one of the diseases that has been most closely defined by genetic arguments. Kelly E. Happe looks at the rhetoric of race with regard to breast cancer to examine the underlying structure of such arguments. In conclusion, Joseph L. Graves, Jr and Michael R. Rose provide a summary of the arguments against the 'bright lines' drawn by racial medicine for the twenty-first century. The question of race has reappeared; the conversation among scholars recognizes the complexity and ambiguity of such categories.

This volume is aimed at examining the claims of these scientific 'bright lines', but also at taking the extraordinary findings of the new genetics seriously. In recent years, modern biological science in the realm of medicine has made breathtaking leaps in the area of genetics and brain imaging that can only be compared to the innovations with regard to endocrinology and infectious diseases at the close of the nineteenth century. The commonplaces associated with those true breakthroughs in our understanding of human biology were clouded by the assumptions of race: the Jews as a 'diabetic' people (a view even held by many Jewish scientists of the time) or the so-called immunity of African Americans to the baneful effects of tertiary syphilis (the premise that the 'liberal' scientists in the horrendous experiments at Tuskegee wished to disprove).[5] Modern genetics has an effect on our self-perception as 'biological entities'. To what degree this reinscribes older fallacies about group identity and establishes them as 'fact' is still very much an issue for debate. This volume is part of that debate.

Sander L. Gilman
Graduate Institute of the Liberal Arts, Emory University

---

5 See Sander L. Gilman, 'Fat as disability: the case of the Jews', *Literature and Medicine*, vol. 23, no. 1, 2004, 46–60; James H. Jones, *Bad Blood: The Tuskegee Syphilis Experiment* (New York: Free Press 1993); and Paul A. Lombardo and Gregory M. Dorr, 'Eugenics, medical education and the public health service: another perspective on the Tuskegee syphilis experiment', *Bulletin of the History of Medicine*, vol. 80, 2006, 291–316.

Blood and stories: how genomics is rewriting race, medicine and human history

PRISCILLA WALD

ABSTRACT   In 2003 Howard University announced its intention to create a databank of the DNA of African Americans, most of whom were patients in their medical centre. Proponents of the decision invoked the routine exclusion of African Americans from research that would give them access to the most up-to-date medical technologies and treatments. They argued that this databank would rectify such exclusions. Opponents argued that such a move tacitly affirmed the biological (genetic) basis of race that had long fuelled racism as well as that the potential costs were not worth the uncertain benefits. Howard University's controversial decision emerges from research in genomic medicine that has added new urgency to the question of the relationship between science and racism. This relationship is the topic of Wald's essay. Scientific disagreements over the relative usefulness of 'race' as a classification in genomic medical research have been obscured by charges of racism and political correctness. The question takes us to the assumptions of population genomics that inform the medical research, and Wald turns to the Human Genome Diversity Project, the new Genographics Project and the 2003 film *Journey of Man* to consider how racism typically inheres not in the intentions of researchers, but in the language, images and stories through which scientists, journalists and the public inevitably interpret information. Wald demonstrates the importance of understanding those stories as inseparable from scientific and medical research. Her central argument is that if we understand the power of the stories we can better understand the debates surrounding race and genomic medicine, which, in turn, can help us make better ethical and policy decisions and be useful in the practices of science and medicine.

In the last week of May 2003 the National Human Genome Center (NHGC) of Howard University announced a plan to create a databank of the DNA of individuals of African descent. The *New York Times* called it 'the nation's largest repository of DNA from African-Americans', and explained that its creation was motivated by a history of racial discrimination in the United States that found expression in disparities of health care. 'We want to make sure', noted the dean of the medical school, Floyd J. Malveaux, that 'as genetics move forward, as information is collected, as data is being mined, that we are part of that process'.[1] With biotechnology widely hailed as the harbinger of a medical revolution, researchers at Howard wanted to ensure that the black population in the United States would have full access to the most up-to-date health care. They viewed the databank, which was projected to house, in five years, DNA samples from 25,000 African-descended individuals, collected mainly from patients at hospitals and clinics associated with Howard's medical school, as crucial to that inclusion. No one involved in the decision was unaware of the risks of such a databank, but its proponents believed that the nation's history of anti-black discrimination and glaring disparities in health care made the countervailing danger of African-American exclusion from the benefits of genomic research more urgent. Arthur L. Holden, president of the First Genetic Trust, a Chicago company chosen to help create the databank, insisted that the only controversial decision would be the refusal to pursue the collection of data.[2]

Critics of the decision conceded the potential usefulness of the information, but worried that it could be misleading and wondered if the benefits were really worth the possible consequences. Genomic research that rested on racial classifications risked reanimating an inaccurate understanding of the biological basis of racial difference, which has been central to racist thought for centuries, as well as underscoring the genetic causes of racially based health disparities at the expense of social and environmental explanations. One of the most prominent critics of the decision, sociologist Troy Duster, expressed concern about other uses of the information collected in such a databank besides medical research and treatment, including forensic racial profiling.[3] The Howard researchers proposed the databank against the backdrop of research concerning the role of genes in disease susceptibility and drug responses, and the development of a drug called BiDil, the first medication to be marketed specifically to a racial group. This research drew its urgency from genomic medicine, but its evidence from the findings of population genomics. As genomic research has become increasingly central to the practice of cutting-edge medicine, debate has centred on whether or not racial classifications offer useful medical information and, if so, with what consequences.

---

1 Andrew Pollack, 'DNA of Blacks to be gathered to fight illness', *New York Times*, 27 May 2003, A1.
2 Ibid.
3 Malcolm Ritter, 'As role of race in research questioned, a DNA databank proposed for Blacks', *Associated Press*, 19 July 2003.

Many scientists have resisted yielding to what they see as social pressures, insisting on the integrity of scientific enquiry and believing that a better understanding of the science will countermand its appropriation for racist arguments. Racism, they insist, in what has become a refrain, is a social problem that has nothing to do with the practice of science. With equal conviction, cultural critics maintain that social assumptions and biases infuse scientific concepts, paradigms and practices; racism is therefore not the result of poorly understood science but is often reproduced unwittingly and against researchers' best intentions. Stuart Hall, for example, cautions 'against extrapolating a common and universal structure to racism' that obscures 'how thoroughly racism is reorganized and rearticulated with the relations of new modes of production'.[4] The idea of 'articulation' in this context conjoins the two primary meanings of the term: the expression of ideas and the formation of connections through flexible joints. With a legacy in Marxist and ideological criticism, the term expresses the structural relationship among disparate things or ideas—for example, labour relations, race and ethnicity, and access to health care—as they are formulated and enacted through specific social practices. Genomic research produces information. Racism is articulated within that information (which is a *product*) through conventions of representation: familiar words and phrases, stock images, plotlines, interpretations and even the classifications that organize research. The archive of those images and expressions as well as the range of discussions about the research, from the scientific and medical literature to the mainstream media and popular culture, comprise the 'stories' of race and genomic medicine. These stories function as a kind of technology: they act instrumentally on the world, making information comprehensible and meaningful, and they constitute as well as produce a body of knowledge.

To understand how genomic research can reproduce racism, it is necessary to understand how racism is articulated through that research as it is practised in the context of particular social formations. The articulation is produced through stories of race and genomic research, which take many forms as they make their way from the scientific community to the general public. Stories about the research reach public consciousness through such controversial decisions as the NHGC databank as well as through the discoveries and innovations emerging from the labs of pharmaceutical companies, universities and federal institutions. Accounts of genomic research offer exciting promises, ranging from new explanations (and treatments) for some of the most feared medical problems, from cancer to avian flu, to new ways of understanding (and managing) human behaviour. They also capture the public imagination with claims of new discoveries that offer insight into the mysteries of human origins and human history, and the

---

4 Stuart Hall, 'Race, articulation, and societies structured in dominance', in Philomena Essed and David Theo Goldberg (eds), *Race Critical Theories* (Oxford: Blackwell 2002), 38–68 (57).

genealogies of individuals as well as groups. The claims and promises fuse in the stories of genomic research broadcast in the mainstream media, and they in turn influence policy and funding decisions and help to shape future research. These stories are fundamental in the production of scientific and medical knowledge and, therefore, as I argue in what follows, attention to them needs to be incorporated into scientific and medical research.

Race and genomic variation

Less than two weeks prior to the public announcement of the databank, the NHGC hosted a workshop, 'Human Genome Variation and "Race"', to address the connections among race and ethnicity, genomic research and human health and medicine. Sponsors of the workshop included the Office of Science of the US Department of Energy, the Irving Harris Foundation, the National Human Genome Research Institute of the National Institutes of Health, and Howard University;[5] selected papers were published in a 2004 supplementary issue of *Nature Genetics*. In their introductory commentary on the volume, Charmaine D. M. Royal and Georgia M. Dunston, both of the NHGC, noted an apparent 'consensus that "race," whether imposed or self-identified, is a weak surrogate for various genetic and nongenetic factors in correlations with health status'.[6] Yet, that 'consensus' belies the diverse claims in the volume.

There is consensus that 'race' has a wide array of definitions, and that it is a complicated term, but the contributors to the special issue show a range of opinions not only about whether, but about when and how 'race' can be a useful category of analysis in medical research. Sarah A. Tishkoff and Kenneth K. Kidd, for example, affirm both that 'knowledge of ancestry can be important clinically and in design of biomedical research studies' and that the 'emerging picture is that populations do, generally, cluster by broad geographic regions that correspond with racial classification'.[7] Joanna L. Mountain and Neil Risch understand 'racial and ethnic categories [as] . . . proxies for a wide range of factors, potentially genetic and nongenetic'. While their concern with the potential misuse of genomic information makes them wary of using racial classifications in genomic research, they maintain that 'an individual's racial or ethnic affiliation will continue to be valuable

5 Ari Patrinos, '"Race" and the human genome' (Sponsor's Foreword), *Nature Genetics*, vol. 36, no. 11s (Supplement), November 2004, S1–S2 (S1).

6 Charmaine D. M. Royal and Georgia M. Dunston, 'Changing the paradigm from "race" to human genome variation', *Nature Genetics*, vol. 36, no. 11s (Supplement), November 2004, S5–S7 (S7).

7 Sarah A. Tishkoff and Kenneth K. Kidd, 'Implications of biogeography of human populations for "race" and medicine', *Nature Genetics*, vol. 36, no. 11s (Supplement), November 2004, S21–S27 (S25–S26).

information in the context of epidemiological research'.[8] Francis S. Collins, by contrast, insists that the weak definitions of 'race' and 'ethnicity' make them 'flawed surrogates for multiple environmental and genetic factors in disease causation, including ancestral geographic origins, socioeconomic status, education and access to health care'. Accordingly, he urges that research 'move beyond these weak and imperfect proxy relationships to define the more proximate factors that influence health care'.[9] Significantly, several of these contributors have taken different positions on this issue either before or since the special issue.[10] The scientific study of race is clearly a vexed topic.[11]

While the contributors do not share a common view of the desired role of race and ethnicity in genomic medical research, they do share a common commitment to the effort to understand the usefulness of genomic research for the health care of individuals and populations, and a concern about the potential misapprehension and misuse of the information that this research generates. The well-known history of atrocities and abuse associated with scientific experimentation generally and, in the twentieth century, of genetics (eugenics) particularly makes race and, more specifically, racism central to this concern. A better understanding of the relationship between racism and the scientific study of 'race' could help to clarify both the problem of the misuse of information and the best way to address it.

Many of the contributors to the special issue, as well as other researchers working in this area, have sought to circumvent the problems raised by 'race' and 'ethnicity' by substituting 'ancestry' and 'population'. Royal and Dunston, for example, follow their rejection of 'race' as a surrogate with the observation that, as we commence this 'new era in molecular medicine, [it] remains to be determined how increasing knowledge of genetic variation in populations will

---

8 Joanna L. Mountain and Neil Risch, 'Assessing genetic contributions to phenotypic differences among "racial" and "ethnic" groups', *Nature Genetics*, vol. 36, no. 11s (Supplement), November 2004, S48–S53 (S52).

9 Francis S. Collins, 'What we do and don't know about "race," "ethnicity," genetics and health at the dawn of the genome era', *Nature Genetics*, vol. 36, no. 11s (Supplement), November 2004, S13–S15 (S13).

10 The difference is most likely a matter of emphasis or even context. Neil Risch, for example, had taken a stronger position on the value of 'race' as a surrogate in a 2002 piece in *Genome Biology* that I will discuss later in this essay. And Francis Collins is depicted, in a piece in the *New York Times Magazine* that appeared in October 2004, as advocating, at least in a limited way, the use of 'race' as a surrogate; see Robin Marantz Henig, 'The genome in black and white (and gray)', *New York Times Magazine*, 10 October 2004, 46–51.

11 For a summary of the field, see Race, Ethnicity and Genetics Working Group, 'The use of racial, ethnic, and ancestral categories in human genetics research', *American Journal of Human Genetics*, vol. 77, no. 4, October 2005, 519–32, and Celeste Condit, 'How culture and science make race "genetic"', *Literature and Medicine*, special issue on 'Genomics and the Arts' (forthcoming). For a discussion of how racism structures the debate itself, see especially Alys Eve Weinbaum, 'Coda: gene/alogies for a new millennium', in *Wayward Reproductions: Genealogies of Race and Nation in Trans-Atlantic Modern Thought* (Durham, NC: Duke University Press 2004), 227–46.

change prevailing paradigms of human health and identity'.[12] Researchers consistently express the hope that the science itself will solve the problem of racism both by showing the common origins and genomic similarities of the human species and by demonstrating the history and mechanisms of human difference. Tishkoff and Kidd insist on the biomedical importance of 'the global distribution of genetic variation' but 'emphasize that the existence of differences, however small, should not be a basis for discrimination'.[13] Yet, as Lisa Gannett has shown, the substitution of 'population' for 'race' dates back to the early work on population genetics in the mid-twentieth century;[14] the concept of 'population' that was articulated in this work, especially by Theodosius Dobzhansky, the founder of the field, absorbed and transformed but did not replace the problematic concept of 'race'.[15] The legacy is evident in

12 Royal and Dunston, 'Changing the paradigm from "race" to human genome variation', S7.
13 Tishkoff and Kidd, 'Implications of biogeography of human populations for "race" and medicine', S26.
14 Lisa Gannett, 'Racism and human genome diversity research: the ethical limits of "population thinking"', *Philosophy of Science*, vol. 68 (Supplement), September 2001, S479–S492.
15 Of particular note is the debate between Dobzhansky and Frank B. Livingstone published as 'On the non-existence of human races' in *Current Anthropology*, vol. 3, no. 3, June 1962, 279–81. Here Livingstone proposed that 'race' be abandoned as a term to describe living populations of human beings on the grounds that biological variation among populations 'does not conform to the discrete packages labeled races' (279). 'Race', he argued, is inaccurate, failing both to correspond to genetic variation and to offer a sufficient explanation for that variation. He was particularly interested in the incompatibility between race and natural selection. Livingstone advocated the substitution of 'clines' for 'races', where 'clines' named gradients of genetic variations among groups that resulted from a variety of factors. Dobzhansky rejected Livingstone's premises, arguing for the biological basis of racial differences and locating the problem of defining 'race' in its status as 'a category of biological classification. ... Discovery of races is a biological problem', he explained, while 'naming races is a nomenclatorial problem' (280). Livingstone, in turn, argued both for the inconsistency of Dobzhansky's definitions of 'race' and for the insupportability of his methodology. 'No science can divorce its concepts, definitions, and theories so completely from its subject matter', he contended, 'so that Dobzhansky's dichotomy between biological and nomenclatorial problems is impossible' (280). Despite radical disagreement over the biology of 'race', however, Dobzhansky and Livingstone shared an interest in avoiding both its ambiguities and its dangers by substituting an alternative nomenclature. I have reproduced this debate here both because of its historical importance and because the terms of this disagreement have (strikingly) continued into the present. Carleton S. Coon's *The Origins of Races* (New York: Alfred A. Knopf 1962) was also an important source in the dissemination of the concept of 'clines'. Like Livingstone and Dobzhansky, he drew on Julian S. Huxley's 'Clines: an auxiliary taxonomic principle', *Nature*, vol. 142, 1938, 219–20. Gianfranco Biondi and Olga Rickards offer a history of the debate in 'The scientific fallacy of the biological concept of race', *Mankind Quarterly*, vol. 42, no. 4, Summer 2002, 355–88. The critical responses to their essay in the same issue of the journal exemplify how the terms of Dobzhansky and Livingstone's debate are being reproduced.

Tishkoff and Kidd's observation about the correspondence of the broad geographical regions that constitute 'populations' and conventional racial classifications.[16]

The solution is not to excise the concept of 'race'. As the seven NHGC authors note in their collaborative piece for the special issue, the

> absence of 'races' does not mean the absence of racism, or the structured inequality based on operationalized prejudice used to deprive people who are deemed to be fundamentally biologically different of social and economic justice. The 'no biological race' position does not exclude the idea that racism is a problem that needs to be addressed.[17]

Duster, perhaps the foremost theorist of race and genomics, is similarly critical of the consortium of scientists who issued the 'Revised UNESCO Statement on Race' in 1995 for their effort to address the problem of racism by declaring 'race' to be a scientifically invalid concept. Racial and ethnic classifications, for Duster, are too deeply 'embedded in the routine collection and analysis of data (from oncology to epidemiology, from hematology to social anthropology, from genetics to sociology)' to be profitably excluded from scientific study.[18] He proposes instead that the study of scientific conceptions of 'race' begins with an understanding of the 'complex interplay of social and biological realities with ideology and myth'.[19] Scientific knowledge, in other words, is invariably situated in social and cultural contexts and must be understood in those terms.

'Race' and 'ethnicity' may or may not be appropriate surrogates for the study of genetic and non-genetic health issues, but they are very much surrogates in the contributions to the special issue as well as other scientific discussions on the topic for a variety of questions concerning the many uses of genomic information. The language of promise and the considerable investments of time and resources have made it difficult to pose questions about the equity, expenditure and distribution that accompany the genomic turn in medicine. The history of racism makes race an especially pressing and visible example of the abuse of scientific information. Racism is not only a problem in its own right, but also a catch-all for the social and cultural

16 I make a similar point about the substitution of 'population' for 'race' in Priscilla Wald, 'Future perfect: genes, grammar and geography', *New Literary History*, vol. 4, no. 31, Autumn 2000, 681–708.

17 S. O. Y. Keita, R. A. Kittles, C. D. M. Royal, G. E. Bonney, P. Furbert-Harris, G. M. Dunston and C. N. Rotimi, 'Conceptualizing human variation', *Nature Genetics*, vol. 36, no. 11s (Supplement), November 2004, S17–S20 (S16).

18 Troy Duster, 'Buried alive: the concept of race in science', in Alan H. Goodman, Deborah Heath and M. Susan Lindee (eds), *Genetic Nature/Culture: Anthropology and Science beyond the Two-Culture Divide* (Berkeley and London: University of California Press 2003), 258–77 (258).

19 Ibid., 259.

inequities that emerge in, and may be exacerbated by, accounts of genomic research.

Race and genomic medicine

Despite disagreements among researchers about how useful 'race' and 'ethnicity' may be as surrogates for genetic and non-genetic health factors, those accounts register an urgency that reinforces a hierarchy of knowledge in which social and cultural enquiry is often cast as naive or even obstructionist. The NHGC's justification for the databank, for example, conveys faith in a medical revolution from which individuals of African descent risk exclusion if they do not take the immediate action represented by the databank. The refusal of a biological basis for 'race' among some of the early population geneticists surfaces in these accounts as evidence of the intrinsic anti-racism of the field. In particular, Richard Lewontin's 1972 article, in which he published the results of a study that demonstrated that genomic variation was significantly greater within than between racial groups, has become the touchstone for discussions of genomic variation. Lewontin declared human 'racial classification ... to be of virtually no genetic or taxonomic significance' and the essay, in which he concluded that 'no justification can be offered for its continuance', is invoked consistently to illustrate the incompatibility of responsible scientific investigation and racism.[20] Against these claims, reports of medical research insist nonetheless that racial and ethnic distinctions offer information that is too important to ignore.

The mainstream media have reproduced this formulation as actively as the specialist literature. A July 2003 *Washington Post* piece on the controversial role of race in clinical drug trials offers a typical example. Drawing on a simplified explanation of Lewontin's point, the author explains that

> recent advances in genetic mapping have all but dismissed race as a biological construct. Race accounts for only a tiny amount of the 0.1 percent genetic variation between one human and [an]other. That means that someone who is considered black, for instance, might have more genes in common with someone who is white rather than someone who is also black.

The explanation is immediately followed by a qualification. 'Yet, on the other hand', notes the writer, 'science also has shown that certain groups share inherited traits, and often similar ailments'.[21] Medicine emerges subtly in

---

20 Richard C. Lewontin, 'The apportionment of human diversity', *Evolutionary Biology*, vol. 6, 1972, 381–98 (397).
21 Ariana Eunjung Cha, 'Race plays role in new drug trials: treatment by genetic origin, ethnicity divides medical profession', *Washington Post*, 28 July 2003, A01.

this formulation as the compelling reason for bringing a biological construction of race back into consideration. Population genomics has all but disproved the biological existence of race, *yet* the correlation between race and health makes the biological underpinnings too important to ignore.

Much of the publicity surrounding the issue resulted, as in the *Washington Post* piece, from reports of a drug produced by NitroMed Inc., a biotech company, to treat heart failure in Blacks. Scientists had founded NitroMed in the mid-1990s to develop nitric oxide-based therapies to treat heart failure. The company acquired the rights to BiDil after the Food and Drug Administration (FDA) had already declined to approve the drug in the absence of an appropriate study; however, a reorganization of the data according to race led to a race-specific study and, eventually, to the long-sought patent.[22] In 2005 BiDil became the first drug marketed specifically to a racial or ethnic group.[23] The research that led to the development and approval of the drug exemplifies the scientific controversy. Critics argue that the race-based study was driven by circumstances that were extraneous to scientific research, that the ambiguous statistics do not justify the claim that the drug is more effective for individuals of African descent, and that the publicity surrounding these findings is irresponsible and market-driven.[24] Whatever its motivation, the publicity certainly invigorated public discussions about the medical relevance of racial and ethnic ancestry.

BiDil, however, did not inaugurate these debates. A *New York Times* piece about the publication of a scientific article on the use of self-identified race and ethnicity as classifications in genomic medical research in a 2002 issue of *Genome Biology* shows the newsworthiness of the topic, independent of specific pharmaceutical developments.[25] The scientific article, 'Categorization of Humans in Biomedical Research: Genes, Race and Disease',[26] presents the response of Stanford population geneticist Neil Risch *et al.* to James F. Wilson *et al.*'s argument for race-blind genomic research.[27] Wilson *et al.* had concluded, in the words of Howard McLeod in an accompanying

22 Pamela Sankar and Jonathan Kahn, 'BiDil: race medicine or race marketing?', *Health Affairs*, Web Exclusive, 11 October 2005.

23 An article in the *New York Times Magazine* in October 2005 helped to publicize both BiDil and the surrounding debate; see Henig, 'The genome in black and white (and gray)'.

24 Sankar and Kahn, 'BiDil'; Jonathan Kahn, 'Getting the numbers right: statistical mischief and racial profiling in heart failure research', *Perspectives in Biology and Medicine*, vol. 46, no. 4, 2003, 473–83.

25 Nicholas Wade, 'Race is seen as real guide to track roots of disease', *New York Times*, 30 July 2002, F1.

26 Neil Risch, Esteban Burchard, Elad Ziv and Hua Tang, 'Categorization of humans in biomedical research: genes, race and disease', *Genome Biology*, vol. 3, no. 7, July 2002, 1–12.

27 James F. Wilson, Michael E. Weale, Alice C. Smith, Fiona Gratix, Benjamin Fletcher, Mark G. Thomas, Neil Bradman and David B. Goldstein, 'Population genetic structure of variable drug response', *Nature Genetics*, vol. 29, no. 3, November 2001, 265–9.

commentary, that 'clusters identified by genotyping ... are far more robust than those identified using geographic and ethnic labels',[28] that, in other words, data from the race-blind study of genetic markers associated with disease yield more useful information than data classified by self-identified race and ethnicity. Risch *et al.* took issue both with Wilson *et al.*'s study and with editorials in scientific publications that drew on it to argue against racial and ethnic classification in genomic medical research. Risch *et al.* disagreed particularly with two positions: the insistence that there is 'no biological basis for race', and the advocacy of 'a "race-neutral" approach' to research in genomic medicine.[29] They maintain, by contrast, that 'from both an objective and scientific (genetic and epidemiologic) perspective there is great validity in racial/ethnic self-categorizations, both from the research and public policy points of view'.[30] Their article, however, does not fully support this conclusion. While Risch *et al.* argue persuasively for the epidemiological usefulness of self-identified race and ethnicity, they do not convincingly present the genetic basis of their claim.

Their argument turns on—and begins to unravel around—the definition of 'biological', for which they offer two possibilities. 'If biological is defined as genetic', they contend, 'then ... a decade or more of population genetics research has documented genetic, and therefore biological, differentiation among the races'.[31] As I have noted, however, there is considerable disagreement among scientists about what the research has documented. Unlike many population geneticists, Risch *et al.* assert that 'two Caucasians are more similar to each other genetically than a Caucasian and an Asian'.[32] To support this claim, they draw on studies in population genomics that, they argue, 'have recapitulated the classical definition of races based on continental ancestry—namely African, Caucasian (European and Middle East), Asian, Pacific Islander (for example, Australian, New Guinean and Melanesian), and Native American' and note that, 'for the purpose of this article, [they] define racial groups on the basis of primary continent of origin ... (with some modifications ...)'.[33] This argument reproduces rather than resolves the ambiguity associated with the relationship of ancestry to race. As many of the participants in the NHGC symposium so forcefully insist, there is no 'classical definition' of 'races'.

'*Self-identified* race and ethnicity' further begs the question of the relationship between biology and culture. As has been widely reported in the mainstream media, the increasing popularity of DNA testing for ancestry

28 Howard L. McLeod, 'Pharmacogenetics: more than skin deep', *Nature Genetics*, vol. 29, no. 3, November 2001, 247–8 (247).

29 Risch *et al.*, 'Categorization of humans in biomedical research: genes, race and disease', 1.

30 Ibid.

31 Ibid., 4.

32 Ibid., 5.

33 Ibid., 3.

has shown that many people are surprised by the results of such tests.[34] Researchers have offered such unanticipated results, in fact, as evidence of how population genomics can dispel the myths of racism by demonstrating how interconnected the human population really is. Self-identification does not necessarily yield the most 'objective and scientific' information about one's genomic profile.

Genomic information is notoriously difficult to interpret even by researchers in the field. The frequency of alleles that mark genetic drift—the the rate of genetic changes resulting from mutations, or divergent alleles, in relatively inbred populations—tells where and when there was a divergence within a group. Those alleles are used to mark ancestry. But, as Michael J. Bamshad and Steve E. Olson note, 'how groups are divided depends on which genes are examined; simplistically put, you might fit into one group based on your skin-color genes but another based on a different character-istic'.[35] The DNA that yields information about one's ancestry—typically mitochondrial and Y-chromosome DNA—in fact tells only part of the story of genetic ancestry. The complexity of nuclear DNA does not yield sufficiently clear information to complete it. Moreover, as Jay Kaufman has pointed out, Risch *et al.*'s study relies on the dismissal of 'intermediate groups', such as 'Hispanic Americans', whom Risch *et al.* acknowledge could 'aggregate genetically with Caucasians, Native Americans, African Americans or form their own cluster' and are therefore 'not easily classified',[36] but the size of those groups attenuates their claims.[37] They are too large to be dismissed as an exception. Intermixture is increasingly the rule.

The other definition of 'biology' Risch *et al.* offer is more compelling, but not genetic. If 'biological is defined by susceptibility to, and natural history of, a chronic disease, then again numerous studies over past decades have documented biological differences among the races'.[38] This definition does not distinguish between environmental and genetic *causes* of the racial and

---

34 *Nightline*, the American nightly news programme, for example, featured a man who had lived fifty years defining himself as 'black' only to learn, through an ancestry test performed recreationally by DNAPrint Genomics, that his DNA revealed Indo-European, East Asian and American Indian, but no African, roots. Once again, that lineage reflects a focus on particular markers, and does not tell the whole story of genetic inheritance, although such qualifications do not typically reach the general public. Moreover, that particularization of a genetic lineage countermands the claim that 'we are all African under the skin'.

35 Michael J. Bamshad and Steve E. Olson, 'Does race exist?', *Scientific American*, vol. 289, no. 6, December 2003, 78–85 (78).

36 Risch *et al.*, 'Categorization of humans in biomedical research', 6–7.

37 Jay Kaufman, 'Race and genomic medicine: false premises, false promises', paper given at a symposium on race and genomics, Duke University, Durham, NC, 3 March 2005.

38 Risch *et al.*, 'Categorization of humans in biomedical research', 4.

ethnic differences that are evident in medical *outcomes*. The persuasive argument here is that self-identified race and ethnicity supply relevant information in the epidemiological study of disease and drug response: they are relevant variables in the study of health outcomes.

Risch *et al.* in fact most insistently invoke race in order to introduce social or environmental factors into an analysis of health outcomes. Citing Wilson *et al.*'s conclusion that race-blind genotyping yields more useful medical information than classification by self-identified 'geographic and ethnic labels', they argue that genetic clustering will 'actually create and/or exacerbate problems associated with genetic inferences based on racial differences'.[39] The reason, they explain, is that genetic clustering risks reducing the explanation for medical outcomes to genomics, failing to take 'environmental risk factors' into account. In other words, self-identified race and ethnicity provide the social and environmental contexts that modify genomic information. This assertion is consistent with the claim that self-identified race and ethnicity are relevant to epidemiological research because those classifications can offer important information about social and environmental risk factors, but not necessarily with the assertion that they have a genetic *basis*.

The public story

Science writer Nicholas Wade found Risch *et al.*'s argument sufficiently important to feature it in the *New York Times*. The image of Risch that he paints in this article is of a heroic scientist who is determined to place research above politics, and strike out against a dangerous political correctness. Thus is the public story created. Quoted in support of Risch's argument, prominent geneticist Stephen O'Brien notes that the effort to invalidate 'race' as a biological concept 'comes from honest and brilliant people who are not population geneticists'.[40] The piece does not explain that it is also population geneticists who most strongly (if not consistently) insist on removing 'race' as a biological category and distinguishing it from 'population'. O'Brien goes on to affirm the sincerity of 'those honest and brilliant people' but remarks:

> What is happening here is that Neil and his colleagues have decided the pendulum of political correctness has taken the field in a direction that will hurt epidemiological assessment of disease in the very minorities the defenders of political correctness wish to protect.[41]

39 Ibid., 7.
40 Quoted in Wade, 'Race is seen as real guide to track roots of disease'.
41 Quoted in ibid.

The charge of 'political correctness' obfuscates the terms of the scientific debate. While Wade includes quotations from population geneticists who argue that race-neutral research yields 'more accurate' information, the piece features Risch, who 'has plunged into an arena where many fear to tread', and gives him the last word.[42] The article concludes with his pronouncement: 'We need to value our diversity rather than fear it. ... Ignoring our differences, even if with the best of intentions, will ultimately lead to the disservice of those who are in the minority.'[43] Wade depicts Risch's opponents, by contrast, as offering not an alternative scientific perspective, but a 'race-side-stepping proposal'.[44]

Pointing an accusatory finger at 'political correctness' not only deflects the scientific dispute, but also ignores the medical importance of the social consequences of racism, measured in health outcomes. Drawing a stark contrast between medical science and social concerns, a distinction that Risch *et al.*'s article itself troubles, that accusation renders social concerns suspect except as they provide epidemiologically useful information. Neither Wade nor Risch *et al.* address what constitutes epidemiologically useful information. Risch *et al.* dismiss potential abuses of genomic information (such as those that fuel racism) as unscientific, arguing

> that identifying genetic differences between races and ethnic groups, be they for random genetic markers, genes that lead to disease susceptibility or variation in drug response, is scientifically appropriate. What is not scientific is a value system attached to any such findings.[45]

But this assertion presumes that science and medicine can be divorced from their social contexts and that information circulates in value-neutral terms. History does not support that presumption, and calling racism 'not scientific' does not address the value system or alleviate the problems—including health outcomes—associated with it.

The social and epidemiological causes of differential health outcomes are exactly the problems that Risch *et al.* most persuasively offer to justify their retention of the categories of 'race' and 'ethnicity'. This suggests an epidemiological (rather than politically correct) reason to consider racism, which includes the potential abuses of the genomic information that emerge from racial and ethnic classifications. If, as Risch *et al.* suggest, race and ethnicity might be factors in medical outcomes (hence, their relevance to

---

42 Ibid. In fact, as I have noted, the thorny question of 'race' has been a topic of concern for population geneticists since the inception of the field (see note 15). And the accusation of political pandering has obscured the scientific disagreement from the outset.
43 Quoted in ibid.
44 Ibid.
45 Risch *et al.*, 'Categorization of humans in biomedical research', 11.

epidemiology), then why should the potential medical consequences of retaining them not also be part of this 'scientific' or, in Risch *et al.*'s words, 'objective' analysis? Calling on the language of 'science' and 'objectivity', Risch *et al.* seem effectively to have set the terms according to which the medical impact of racism is a factor only in epidemiological assessment and not in the analysis of health inequities. *Racism*, it seems, as much as race, affects health outcomes; potentially racist uses of racially classified genetic data could have such outcomes and therefore should be factored into these debates *as medically relevant* and not dismissed as 'politically correct'.

Taking racism into account does not mean refusing to collect and classify data in medical research according to race and ethnicity. On the contrary, those classifications provide important epidemiological information, as Risch *et al.* maintain, about the impact of social and environmental factors—including socio-economic inequities and cultural biases—on the health of individuals and groups. As Troy Duster argues, the way to 'recognize, engage, and clarify the complexity of the interaction between *any* taxonomies of race and biological, neurophysiological, society, and health outcomes' is to consider 'how science studies deploy the concept of race'.[46] The story of how biotechnology is revolutionizing medicine has put genomic research very much into public consciousness and has made genetic explanations of health disparities among individuals and especially groups the 'default position'.[47] Distinguishing between genomic and social and environmental factors in disease susceptibility and drug response is notoriously difficult, especially since, as Keita *et al.* note, 'some environmental influences can be so subtle and occur so early in life as to be missed ... '.[48] Yet, that distinction determines how researchers and practitioners understand and address the problem of health disparities. 'Race' and 'ethnicity' are very different as surrogates for genomics and for social and environmental factors in the assessment of health outcomes, which is why the larger stories in which the research is embedded are scientifically and medically as well as socially relevant.

Neither Wade nor Risch *et al.* address the complexity of the information that is emerging from population genomics. The markers currently associated with genomic ancestry, as I have noted, tell only a small part of the story both of an individual's genealogy and of the fluidity of populations over time. The category of 'mixed-race' individuals is growing exponentially as are the number of markers that researchers are discovering. 'Populations' are overlapping and variable. Genotypes and phenotypes, moreover, are often at odds, leading to mischaracterization by 'self-identifying' individuals as well as researchers. Skin pigmentation, for example, results from geographical factors that do not necessarily correlate to genomic similarity,

46 Duster, 'Buried alive', 259.
47 Keita *et al.*, 'Conceptualizing human variation', S19.
48 Ibid.

and different alleles can be responsible for common medical conditions. The medical annals tell tragic stories of misdiagnoses of sickle cell disease or cystic fibrosis because the patient's 'race' did not conform to assumptions about the genetic dispositions of the disease, and popular media in the form of television series have picked up on these stories.[49] Classifications can affect the interpretation of the data. The statistical difference that ostensibly appeared when the BiDil research data were classified by race, for example, could lead to assumptions that would result in a doctor's prescribing the drug when it would be ineffective or failing to prescribe it when it would be useful.

Concern about the racist consequences attendant on race-based genomic research seems to have made some inroads even among the staunchest advocates of the research. The position that Mountain and Risch take evinces a departure from, or at least modification of, Risch *et al.*'s claims in the earlier article. Noting that 'our lack of understanding of the etiology of many complex traits means that racial and ethnic labels remain useful in epidemiological and clinical settings', Mountain and Risch recognize 'the potential for furthering racism by discussing race and genetics together in a scientific context', and therefore 'might seek to eliminate the use of racial categories in these contexts'.[50] Yet, their reasoning suggests a capitulation to the very 'side-stepping' of which Risch is critical in Wade's article rather than the kind of structural analysis that Duster advocates. Mountain and Risch follow their claim with the assertion that 'current health disparities' and the assumption 'that our society values the goal of understanding the underlying basis of those disparities' justify 'the continued use of labels in epidemiological research and clinical practice ... '[51] Their endnotes send the reader to Risch *et al.*'s earlier 'Categorization of Humans in Biomedical Research' as well as to a concurring piece, E. G. Burchard *et al.*'s 'The Importance of Race and Ethnic Background in Biomedical Research and Clinical Practice'.[52] The nature of the research itself does not seem to be in question.

49 The television series *Chicago Hope*, for example, included an episode about a white woman who was dismissed by medical staff as crazy when she insisted she was suffering from sickle cell disease, but who, when she was finally tested, turned out to be correct. Richard S. Garcia has publicized a similar case of misdiagnosis in 'The misuse of race in medical diagnosis', *Chronicle of Higher Education*, 9 May 2003, B15. See also Lynn B. Jorde and Stephen P. Wooding, 'Genetic variation, classification and "race"', *Nature Genetics*, vol. 36, no. 11s (Supplement), November 2004, S28–S33.

50 Mountain and Risch, 'Assessing genetic contributions to phenotypic differences among "racial" and "ethnic" groups', S52.

51 Ibid.

52 Esteban González Burchard, Elad Ziv, Natasha Coyle, Scarlett Lin Gomez, Hua Tang, Andrew J. Karter, Joanna L. Mountain, Eliseo J. Pérez-Stable, Dean Sheppard and Neil Risch, 'The importance of race and ethnic background in biomedical research and clinical practice', *New England Journal of Medicine*, vol. 348, no. 12, March 2003, 1170–5.

Mountain and Risch, like most of the other participants in the NHGC symposium, concede the complexity of the information that emerges from population genomics, although the participants vary in the emphasis they put on that complexity. Royal and Dunston, in fact, call attention to the 'scientific focus of the inaugural meeting in the *Human Genome Variation and "Race"* series'—and therefore to the special issue that it spawned—and concede that a 'substantial portion of the ongoing dialog on this issue has been devoted to the glaring medical and societal implications, often glossing over the ambiguous science that underlies many of these implications'.[53] The information that emerges from population genomics about the 'meaning' of human genomic variation and its relevance to the practice of medicine is central to an understanding of how race and racism articulate to genomic research. Population genomics supplies the information and categories—and, in effect, constitutes the underlying story—of 'race' and genomic medicine. That story needs to be part of the discussion.

The genomic story of human diversity

If medicine brings urgency to the question of the biological basis of race, human history brings drama and scope. Retelling the story of human migrations is in fact the chief aim of the field of population genomics, even if medicine offers the most fertile ground for the application of its insights. As one of the most prominent figures in the field, Luigi Luca Cavalli-Sforza, explains, population genomics offers a way to resolve the chaos of cultural definitions: 'human populations', he observes, 'are hard to define in a way that is both rigorous and useful because human beings group themselves in a bewildering array of sets, some of them overlapping, all of them in a state of flux'.[54] In his view, population genomics can sort out the categories and replace social chaos with scientific order; it can, that is, tell a more orderly story about genomic information.

Population geneticists chart the movements and migrations of people by measuring genetic drift. The frequency of alleles can offer information about when a group branched off from the 'family tree'. Allelic frequency is like a photograph of a population, fixing it in—and defining it by—a particular moment in time. Over long periods of time, populations are fluid, as early population geneticists sought to acknowledge with the concept of 'clines', or gradual shifts between populations. DNA, as Bamshad and Olson observe,[55] records a person's membership in any number of populations, which vary

53 Royal and Dunston, 'Changing the paradigm from "race" to human genome variation', S6.
54 Luigi Luca Cavalli-Sforza, 'Genes, peoples and languages', *Scientific American*, vol. 265, November 1991, 104–11 (104).
55 Bamshad and Olson, 'Does race exist?'.

according to the source of the DNA and the markers that are under consideration. The account of a person's 'ancestry' marks a decision to begin his or her descent at a particular historic and geographic point and on the basis of selected information. The technologies used to chronicle human migration can equally generate a picture of distinct biological populations. The same data can yield—have yielded—different stories. Yet, the concept of a (genetic) diaspora suggests that a fixed conception of the group can transcend the historical and geographical particularities. There is an inherent tension in population genomics between the fluidity of the concept of a population that population geneticists characteristically underscore, and the methodology and models of the discipline that seem designed to discover its fixity. Genomic information emerges, and is interpreted, through that tension.

The social categories, moreover, have been tenacious. While populations may not conform exactly to contemporary racial taxonomies, they reflect the evolution of human differences that more or less map on to the familiar categories, not only in popular discussions but, as several of the contributions to the NHGC symposium published in the special issue of *Nature Genetics* attest, in many scientific accounts as well. The story makes all the difference. The contradictions are evident in the urgent claim with which the editors preface the special issue that 'unless we discuss human genome variation, we will all miss the emerging story of who we are and where we come from'.[56] Although they explicitly advocate abandoning 'race' in favour of 'human genome variation', they do not consider how 'genome variation' has itself posed thorny questions about classification. The formulation implicit in '*the* emerging story' eludes the multiple (and contested) stories that are in fact emerging from the data. There are, that is, many stories about human migration and variation that could be supported by the scientific research as well as by data in other fields. This statement, moreover, presumes a coherent 'we' and defers the question of who has the authority to write its history. The stories about genomic information influence what is seen and, conversely, what is not seen. They have material consequences, since they affect funding, policy and even research and health outcomes. The contest over the emerging stories is therefore medically as well as socially relevant.

That contest was at the heart of the controversies surrounding the Human Genome Diversity Project (HGDP), which grew out of the critique, issued by Cavalli-Sforza and others, of the homogeneity of the Human Genome Project (HGP). He and his colleagues were—and remain—determined, as he explains in the April 2005 issue of *Nature Genetics*, to provide 'a resource that is aimed at promoting worldwide research on human genetic diversity, with the ultimate goal of understanding how and when patterns of diversity

56 'The unexamined population' (Editorial), *Nature Genetics*, vol. 36, no. 11s (Supplement), November 2004, S3. The claim can be read as a tacit defence of the field of (human) population genomics, in which human genome variation has always been the central focus.

were formed'.[57] The goals of the HGDP were articulated and shaped in a series of symposia in the early 1990s that addressed the scientific, ethical and anthropological issues involved in chronicling the history of human migration by collecting and studying the DNA of isolated population groups worldwide.[58] From the outset, the project reflected an overriding interest in reconstructing a more accurate history of genetic diversity and human migration patterns and the conviction that the DNA of relatively isolated—'indigenous'—populations contained the most pertinent, and most easily studied, information. The contention that these populations were on the verge of cultural (and biological) extinction lent urgency to the project. While its proponents cited the medical benefits of the information that would be gathered, those benefits were not foremost in the original justification for the research.[59]

Cavalli-Sforza and his colleagues were surprised to encounter charges of racism as the project increasingly gained public notice. Objections from indigenous groups worldwide to the assumptions and nature of the research as well as to its feared consequences—what they termed 'biocolonialism'—helped to halt work on the project. From the perspective of a decade, Cavalli-Sforza summarizes the objections he encountered as 'the fear that indigenous people might be exploited by the use of their DNA for commercial purposes ("bio-piracy")' and the anxiety 'expressed', as he puts it, 'by naïve observers' that the data generated by the HGDP would fuel '"scientific racism" ... despite the fact that half a century of research into human variation has supported the opposite point of view—that there is no scientific basis for racism'.[60] The planning document for the HGDP included among the list of practical applications for the research that it would 'help to combat the widespread popular fear and ignorance of human genetics and [would] make a significant contribution to the elimination of racism'.[61] The scientists involved in the project believed that understanding the nature of human genomic variation was the best way to see the unity of the human species. From their point of view, they had only good intentions, but

57 Luigi Luca Cavalli-Sforza, 'The Human Genome Diversity Project: past, present and future', *Nature Genetics*, vol. 6, April 2005, 333–40 (333).
58 Ibid.
59 I have written about the response to the HGDP in Wald, 'Future perfect'. The most extensive treatment of the history and critique of the project is Jenny Reardon, *Race to the Finish: Identity and Governance in an Age of Genomics* (Princeton, NJ and Oxford: Princeton University Press 2004). See also Jonathan Marks, ' "We're going to tell these people who they really are": science and relatedness', in Sarah Franklin and Susan McKinnon (eds), *Relative Values: Reconfiguring Kinship Studies* (Durham, NC: Duke University Press 2001), 355–83 and, for a discussion of the arbitrariness of genomic classification, Jonathan Marks, *What It Means to Be 98% Chimpanzee: Apes, People, and Their Genes* (Berkeley: University of California Press 2002).
60 Cavalli-Sforza, 'The Human Genome Diversity Project', 333.
61 Quoted in Steve E. Olson, 'The genetic archaeology of race', *Atlantic Monthly*, vol. 287, no. 4, April 2001, 69–74, 76, 78–80 (73).

Cavalli-Sforza's current understanding of the problem manifests the same logic that leads researchers to 'side-step' race in their medical studies; he locates the problem in the difficulties surrounding the question of 'race' and fails to address the concerns articulated by the critics of the project. He simply declares racism (as opposed to race) to be scientifically baseless. Even Steve Olson, in an *Atlantic Monthly* piece about the conflict that is sympathetic to Cavalli-Sforza, concedes that, for his belief that 'if people understood genetics, they couldn't possibly be racists', Cavalli-Sforza 'must certainly be judged naïve'.[62]

The most sustained critique of the work has come from the Indigenous Peoples Council on Biocolonialism (IPCB), which emerged from indigenous opposition to the HGDP.[63] More complex than Cavalli-Sforza's summary suggests, the IPCB's charges address the inscription of his proposed genomic research in the social and economic inequities that reflect centuries of colonization in which resources, defined broadly to include human labour and human being, were exploited and populations were oppressed often to the point of annihilation. That exploitation can take many forms and even has a history relevant to genomic research, as exemplified in the case of the Hagahai. In 1984 the Hagahai people of Papua New Guinea requested medical assistance for the many diseases that were afflicting them. An anthropologist who made contact with the group took blood samples for diagnostic purposes, but when medical researchers discovered unusual immunological properties in the blood of many Hagahai, they used the samples for research and even patented a cell line derived from the DNA of one man. While the controversial patent was withdrawn, the cell line established from his DNA remains available for research purposes. The case raises questions that are relevant to the HGDP in terms both of motivation and of control over the information: who is conducting the research and for what ends? To what uses will the resulting information be put? Who will profit? These questions involve more than money. They express the unequal relationship between the groups: the group in power not only determines how the information will be used, but also the kinds of stories that will be told about it and the material consequences they will generate.

62 Ibid., 80.
63 The earliest organizational opposition came from the Rural Advancement Foundation International (RAFI), a Canadian-based group that had previously concentrated on corporations' exploitation of developing world farmers (Olson, 'The genetic archaeology of race'). Objections to the HGDP and its subsequent incarnations have varied, ranging from a specific critique of the nature of the project to broad-based opposition to genomic research and biotechnology generally in all of their forms. Cavalli-Sforza does not distinguish among the objections, dismissing them all with the explanation: 'There are some people who hate biology. ... Or they hate humanity' (quoted in Meredith F. Small, 'First soldier of the gene wars', *Archaeology*, vol. 59, no. 3, May 2006, 46–51 (51)). My own concern in this essay is with the specific critique of the biocolonialism of the HGDP and its offshoots.

The concerns raised by the IPCB are both cultural and socio-economic. Exploitation of resources, they argue, is not limited to financial profit. They also underscore a fundamental clash in world-view between Euroamerica and indigenous cultures that includes differences in spiritual beliefs and in the understanding of property. While it is not only across cultures that some of the practices associated with genomic research might constitute 'a violation of ... cultural and ethical mandates',[64] Euroamerican scientists are less likely to understand the nature of those beliefs held by indigenous communities. And a difference in the conception of property complicates the consent that is requisite for research conducted on human subjects.[65] The IPCB maintains that 'the protocols, rooted in Euro-american thought, [that] assume that the individual has the right to sell or give away anything that is their own ... is in conflict with indigenous notions of group rights'.[66] Certain kinds of knowledge may not be alienable in all cultures, or may belong to the group rather than to an individual. Differing conceptions of property are part of the particularly vexed history of Euroamerican and indigenous relations, since they were used to justify Euroamerican dispossession and colonization of indigenous peoples in the New World. The issue is especially relevant and pressing in genomic research, which is primarily concerned with information about the group rather than about individuals.

Critiques of the project have also questioned the motivation for expending resources on data collection—cell lines for a genomic museum—rather than on other kinds of aid to groups that might address the problems they face, as in the case of the Hagahai. The individualized health care that is the goal of genomic medicine is considerably more relevant for the health problems of Euroamericans than for many of the indigenous populations studied by the HGDP, in which people are dying from treatable diseases such as malaria and measles. The research itself, in so far as it widens the information and technology gaps between wealthy and impoverished nations and communities, can contribute to the social and economic inequities that have created the conditions that threaten the existence of these groups in the first place. The ostensible inevitability of tribal extinction with which the HGDP justified their research, for example, obscures the social and political causes of the problems faced by indigenous peoples—the worldwide inequities and their environmental expressions—that are not inevitable. The language of inevitability, in other words, can cloud the analyses of the problem and forestall the possibility of social change.

---

64 IPCB, 'Indigenous people, genes and genetics: what indigenous people should know about biocolonialism. A primer and a resource guide', June 2000, available on the IPCB website at www.ipcb.org/publications/primers/htmls/ipgg.html (viewed 21 July 2006).
65 Reardon, *Race to the Finish*.
66 IPCB, 'Indigenous people, genes and genetics'.

Cavalli-Sforza and his colleagues do not see how the revolutionary promise of biotechnology, and in particular population genomics, can exacerbate the racism, poverty and other structural inequities that they hope their research will help to abolish. One problem is that they do not acknowledge the impact of the stories through which their research is articulated. As a result, they continue unwittingly to reproduce the problems. Although they lost their federal funding and were forced to abandon the HGDP, it has been reincarnated, with funding from the National Geographic Society, IBM and the Waitt Family Foundation, in the Genographic Project, which was announced in April 2005, the same month in which Cavalli-Sforza's piece on the HGDP appeared in *Nature Genetics*. There have been some changes that register the effort to profit from the critiques—notably, the concerted attempt to involve representatives of indigenous communities more fully in the research project—but the basic contours and storyline of the project remain the same. Cavalli-Sforza, who chairs the advisory board of the new project,[67] continues to defend the HGDP, insisting that it was unfairly criticized and misunderstood, and other public relations ventures attest to an intention to market the present project more effectively to the general public.

Human history and the drama of genomic research

Among the most successful public outreach ventures is a documentary film, *Journey of Man: The Story of the Human Species*, directed by Clive Maltby and hosted by Spencer Wells, a former postdoctoral student of Cavalli-Sforza. The film, which premièred on PBS in January 2003, dramatizes the project of chronicling human history through genomic research. Wells offers rudimentary science lessons in which he explains how he and his colleagues have deduced human migration routes based on the frequency of genetic markers found in Y-chromosome DNA—hence the journey of *man*—as he follows the migratory routes that he posits. National Geographic meets the HGDP in this film, which features Wells's trip around the globe and his meetings with the members of indigenous groups whose DNA forms the basis of the study. In *The Journey of Man: A Genetic Odyssey*, a book published in 2002 as a companion to the documentary, Wells concedes that 'science can sometimes run roughshod over cultural beliefs' and offers his 'hope that this book might be a small step towards changing the field [of population genomics] into what it really is—a collaborative effort between people around the world who are interested in their shared history'.[68] Wells works to dramatize that collaboration in the documentary, but the language, images and

67 Small, 'First soldier of the gene wars', 51.
68 Spencer Wells, *The Journey of Man: A Genetic Odyssey* (Princeton, NJ: Princeton University Press 2002), xvi.

narrative of the film tell a story that in fact exemplifies the concerns of the anti-biocolonialism movement. *Journey of Man* demonstrates how unexamined assumptions can surface in the story through which genomic information is interpreted and presented.

The language of discovery dominates the film. The advertising copy on the DVD captures the tone in its summary of the film:

> There was a time—not so long ago—when the human species numbered only a few thousand and their world was a single continent: Africa. Then something happened. A small group left their African homeland on a journey into an unknown, hostile world. Against impossible odds, these extraordinary explorers not only survived but went on to conquer the earth. Their story can finally be told through the science of genetics.

It identifies Wells as 'part of a team that has been re-writing history. He has been disentangling this epic story from evidence all people carry with them—in their DNA—inherited from those ancient travelers'. Wells *disentangles* rather than *writes* that story, which means that he discovers a story that is already there. Early in the film, he pricks his finger, and the camera moves in for an extreme close-up of a drop of his blood, as Wells describes its content as 'the greatest history book ever written'. The story that Wells is telling is written in the blood and 'discovered' in Cavalli-Sforza's lab. Wells acknowledges neither that he is telling one among many possible stories about the data, nor that the Y-chromosome offers only a partial record of ancestry. He is not telling—and cannot tell—the whole story of human migration.

Wells consistently reiterates an explicit message of human connection, but a familiar developmental hierarchy pervades the language and images. The story he tells begins with the heroism and conceptual sophistication of the first group of modern human beings who left Africa. He explains that the audience of the film descends from them, while his story begins with 'the few survivors they left behind, the San Bushmen'. The visual and narrative features of the film implicitly construct the San as the relics from whom the rest of humanity has evolved, although Wells does not explain that the genomic data cannot definitively confirm that claim. The film freezes the San in genomic time, depicting them as the most direct biological link to—the 'brothers and sisters' of—the original people who made the journey, while 'we' (the audience) are the 'distant cousins' of both. By the end of the initial scene, Wells has begun to refer to the San as 'our living ancestors'. A visual refrain that punctuates the film underscores their role. With each new stage in the journey, Wells invites the viewer to 'walk in the footsteps of our ancestors'. The phrase is accompanied by the superimposed image of 'primitive' people, whose dress and bearing, as they have been established by the film, identify them as San. The monochromatic images are elongated and distorted; the focus projects these diaphanous, spectral figures walking across beaches and deserts out of—and into—a mythic past.

Implicit in the image is the inevitability of their extinction: the ancestors must move on, leaving only the traces of their DNA in the genomes of their descendants and the laboratories of the HGDP in its subsequent incarnations. Modernization and cultural intermingling is recast in the film as a biological extinction that justifies the project as it underscores the impending extinction of the San people. 'Their numbers are dwindling', Wells intones. 'Soon they could be gone entirely. We came none too soon.' The proleptic nostalgia—nostalgia, that is, for a time that is not yet past—certifies as it laments their passing. Their way of life consigns them to a different—and a distant—time. One of the men in the scene thanks Wells for the information that he brings but, as the film makes clear, that information is only evidence of their inscription in a story for which they form the backdrop and in which their passing into myth seems almost to require their departure from the present. Their disappearance is intrinsic to the story that has already been written—literally—in blood.

While the collaboration that Wells espouses depends on a respectful integration of world-views, the film continually recasts indigenous and western knowledge as a distinction between story and science, and genomic knowledge emerges at the top of a hierarchy, as a corrective to the current wisdom of both indigenous tradition and archaeological evidence. Following 'the genetic trail' from Africa to Australia, Wells respectfully demonstrates the information that archaeology can reveal, but he shows its limitations when archaeology can offer no insight into how human beings first got to Australia. Next he turns to the oral culture of the Australian aboriginal songlines to see if there is any evidence of a migration, but the journey they describe does not originate in Africa. Only genomic information can definitively (as he represents it) chronicle human migration routes and tell the story of human history.

A low angle shot of Wells looming in the Australian desert embodies the perspective of the film. Where Wells means to enact collaboration, he consistently displays the explanatory superiority of his methods and his information, as in his interaction with Greg Inibla Goodbye Singh, 'an aboriginal artist from Queensland'. Singh's refusal to accept DNA evidence about his ancestors' African origins over the information in the songlines occasions Wells's performance of his sensitivity to the indigenous concerns and respect for an indigenous world-view. 'It's complicated to explain', Wells begins, simply and off camera. The focus remains on Singh as Wells explains that what he would like Singh 'to think about the DNA stories we're telling is that they are that: they are DNA stories. That's our version as Europeans of how the world was populated and where we all trace back to. That's our story line.' The camera begins to pan right as Wells slowly comes into view, continuing his explanation: 'We use science to tell us about that because we don't have the sense of direct continuity our ancestors didn't pass down as stories.' Wells works hard in this scene to show his respect for Singh's tradition and even uses the analogy between the songlines and the DNA stories—which he calls the resurrection of 'a global songline' in his book[69]—to articulate his hope for collaboration. But his garbled diction betrays his discomfort with his explanation. To Singh he concedes: 'We've lost [the ancestral stories] and we have to go out and find them, and we use science, which is a European way of looking at the world, to do that.' Although he moves rhetorically towards an acknowledgement that his interpretation is one way of telling the story of descent, the film continually distinguishes between 'science' and 'story'. Singh's traditional *stories* lead him to question Wells's assertion that Australians originated in Africa, but Wells's *science* has established the truth of the claim.

While Wells speaks, the camera is still. He is shot in profile, looking, presumably, at Singh and framed by a large rock, some trees and a halo of light. Wells has already established the mystical pull of the land in a conversation with Roy Kennedy, a descendant of the Mungo people, whose affective knowledge makes the desolate site of an archaeological dig feel, in Wells's words, 'like home'. Kennedy confirms his deeply felt connection with the land, as the film displays the preparation and enactment of what is depicted as a traditional ceremony. In the terms of the film, Kennedy's sense of connection to a particular place is inscribed within the world-view of a backward-looking, ritualistic and static culture and implicitly distinguished from the mobility that characterizes western modernity. Although less forceful than Singh, Kennedy, too, insists on his belief that his ancestors are 'from here'.

Considering the critique of the IPCB, the interchange with Singh is crucial. 'You guys don't need that', explains Wells, referring to his research. 'You've got your own stories.' Singh readily assents, as Wells nods sympathetically. A cut to a close-up of Singh, who again strongly affirms his belief in the aboriginal oral tradition, displays his resistance. Wells responds, lamenting, over a cut to a shot of the ocean that dissolves into lab notes: 'This really isn't going very well. Tradition rarely sits well with cutting-edge science.' Relegating the songlines to 'tradition', he contrasts them with the certainty of science, which has established the pattern of migration. The remaining question is the routes human beings took when they left Africa.

'Let's go see if we can make history', Wells proposes, leaving the aborigines to their time warp and heading to India to find the 'elusive Australian marker' through which he claims that he can chronicle the route Africans took to Australia. He calls this marker—an allele present in Australians, but not in Africans—the 'missing link', a term he misleadingly transfers to the individual who carries the allele. Wells significantly over-simplifies the science of this claim, passing over other possible explanations

69 Ibid.

for the presence of the allele; his subsequent discovery of the 'missing link'—visually displayed by the face of the man who carries the allele—suggests that population genomics is rewriting the narrative not only of human migration, but also of human evolution.[70] These discoveries, in other words, constitute a scientific revolution.

Multiple migrations require Wells to choose how he will narrate simultaneous or overlapping migration events, but the language of discovery obscures those choices. Wells consistently reminds viewers that he is following the trail dictated by research, and he does not acknowledge the choices involved in researchers' interpretations of the data or in filmmakers' sense of the drama of the story. One such choice is evident when Wells introduces his own genealogy. At this point, his narration manifests the temporal tangle of population genomics, in which the language of relationality (the *family of man*) oscillates between connection and distinction. While 'we' are all descended from the San, Wells's *own* ancestors, he explains, are from Northern Europe. 'The story gets a little more personal here', he confesses, standing in a forest in France. The shift to the 'personal' brings a change in temporal focus. From the story of a connection to a distant past in Africa, it has become a story about a rupture from that past: the discrete population from which Wells descends *begins* in Northern Europe. Ironically, the personal connection to place brings him rhetorically closer to the point of view expressed by Kennedy and Singh, who insist on the origins of *their* ancestry in Australia. As Wells explains, his

70 Craig Venter makes a similar implicit claim in his recent project that retraces Darwin's routes while doing wide-scale genomic sampling of the flora and fauna. I am grateful to Robert Cook-Deegan for his timely and succinct explanation of the possibilities that Wells does not allow, including the possible mobility of the ancestors from whom the individual inherited the allele, the uncertainties of ancestry (unknown liaisons in more recent history between individuals of different ancestry), even new and coincidental mutations. The story Wells tells, in other words, is one among a range of possibilities. A scene in the film that features Wells's meeting with another of his 'missing links', this one from Central Asia, demonstrates the slipperiness of the language. Wells reports his discovery of an 'ancient marker'—or 'spelling mistake'—that chronicles the ancestry of Europeans in Central Asia, which he calls 'the nursery of mankind'. The term 'missing link' superimposes one kind of evolutionary narrative on to another and turns the man in question—not just his ancestor—into the missing link. The use of language in this scene is misleading for viewers unfamiliar with the science. 'Missing link' suggests a prior stage of evolution in common parlance. Wells potentially creates further confusion when he refers to the man as a 'genetic giant in history', as though the accident of his genetic lineage is an achievement. The information his blood gives to the researchers makes him special, and Wells congratulates him repeatedly on his 'very important blood'. Nor does Wells correct him when, in response to his explanation of the 'meaning' of this marker, the man smiles, thanks him and observes, 'that means my blood is pure'. No one with even a passing familiarity with the language of eugenics could fail to hear a chilling resonance in the discussion of the purity of blood, and it is surprising that Wells chose to leave the comment in the film without any correction or explanation.

ancestors represent a small branch of the tree. While not inconsistent, the alternative temporalities represent two different ways of telling the story of descent. The narration literally *makes* the difference, and Wells unwittingly slips back and forth between them.

With the move to Northern Europe, the film becomes increasingly self-conscious about the science of 'race' and phenotypic distinction. The scene initiates the greatest concentration of scientific 'experts', talking heads who detail the climatological changes that probably motivated the migrations and explain the evolutionary selection behind the mutations that resulted in a change of skin colour and body type. Against a black-and-white (mythic) background in which a dark-skinned 'native' is engaged in spearfishing, Wells notes that geological changes attendant upon the Ice Age isolated this population, resulting in distinctive alterations in such features as hair colour, height and nose shape: features, in other words, that are traditionally associated with 'race'. Subtly, but deliberately, the film offers this scientific explanation of phenotypic difference in response to the charges that this research fosters racism. But the visual and narrative logic of the film undercuts those intentions, as it reaffirms a developmental narrative of ancestry.

The scientific explanations culminate in a French village where a group of men is playing boule. 'Today', intones Wells in voice-over, 'people with European ancestors, like me and these French boule players, look pretty different from our distant relatives'. A series of frames featuring representatives from several of the indigenous groups he has been tracking follows to illustrate the differences. These people, all contemporaries, become the 'distant relatives' of Wells and the French boule players in the logic of the film. The most obvious difference, of course, is skin colour—the film presumes that the audience will all see physical resemblance in the same way—and, while Wells does not use the term 'ancestor', the film has already established the visual vocabulary of a developmental hierarchy and a temporality that is summoned by the photographs of these 'primitive' peoples. During the display of this series, moreover, Wells explains the dramatic change in life skills that transpired as 'our ancestors' made the long and arduous journey to Northern Europe.

The ambiguous phrase 'our ancestors' has by now come to mean the immediate forebears of Europeans, and his invocation interpolates his presumed audience in that group. A close-up of the boule playing, a leisure activity that marks an advanced civilization, suggests a comparison with the ritual activities in which the indigenous groups depicted in the film are engaged. Once again the indigenous groups featured in the film become the living ancestors who herald human development in the West. The scene in the French village is in fact a scientific detour, and temporal forecasting, in the narrative of the film; the genetic trail follows the more 'isolated populations' of 'indigenous' groups, and Wells moves back to Central Asia where he again picks up the genetic trail that eventually culminates in Canyon de Chelly, a sacred site of the Navajo people.

In the penultimate scene of the film, Wells stages the collaboration he has been promising throughout. The IPCB critique looms over the meeting with the representatives of 'an ancient tribe', the Navajo. A conciliatory Wells concedes that he 'wanted to tell them about the genetic trail that had led [him] to them, but [he] soon learned that they had migration stories of their own'. Letty, the one woman in the scene, and the only female 'indigenous' interlocutor in the film, greets him with the assurance that 'we are glad to share our *information* about our place here'. She stresses the word 'information', and it is repeated several times in the scene. But Wells's chief interlocutor is Phil Bluehouse, whose advocacy of a return to Navajo traditions in issues ranging from Navajo law enforcement and medicine to environmental restoration has made him both a celebrity and a logical representative in the Navajo community. Bluehouse picks up the challenge that Greg Singh, the Australian aboriginal artist, had also issued, when he questions Wells's use of the word 'myth'. 'Why do you call something that a people tell you a myth as opposed to an experience that they had and relive ... over and over?', he asks. *Myth*, he explains, is a 'substandard event that does not have any relevance'.

This moment stages the most direct and pointed challenge to Wells that anyone has offered. Where Singh had insisted on his belief in the aboriginal story of origins, Bluehouse turns the focus on Wells, calling attention to his language and the point of view it betrays. The question asks Wells to consider stories as experiential and important to collective identity rather than simply as evidence of uninterrogated belief systems. It underscores the discrepancy between the language of 'story' and 'creation' through which Wells explains his research and the framework in which he actually understands it. But Wells does not follow through on the insight, responding, as he has throughout the film, with the explanation that he is a scientist and he relies on 'evidence'. For him, the struggle is between science and myth, and he does not consider the formative power of stories: that he, too, is a storyteller whose 'information' reflects the choices he has made in the interpretation of his data. While he politely acknowledges Bluehouse's objection that 'myth' is a dismissive term, his self-congratulatory voice-over—'I'm getting pretty good at this'—suggests that the scene is not included as a moment of introspection or collaboration, but as a demonstration of the superiority of scientific explanation. Bluehouse does not contest the science, the evidence or the conclusions of Wells's story; he challenges his language. Wells does not hear the difference, and that is precisely the problem with the film.

Bluehouse, however, accepts the explanation, and his acquiescence marks indigenous support of the project. The scene turns on his eager response to Wells's claims about the genetic lineage of North American indigenous peoples that leads from Central Asia to the Americas. 'Looking at a book from people from Central Asia', Bluehouse quips, 'I saw my cousin Emmett and Abraham and Auntie Grandma Buggs, and I said, "My God, I got family over there in Central Asia."' It is Bluehouse, rather than Wells, who ultimately makes the point 'that somehow we're finally ... acknowledging one another from the scientific realm and the traditional realm'. The ostensible response to the IPCB critique, in other words, comes in the final words of a Navajo man, who tacitly reinforces the point of the film and of the renovated diversity project.

'A desire for cultural privacy, perhaps combined with the suspicion that the scientific results may not agree with their own beliefs', acknowledges Wells in his book,

> is leading more and more indigenous groups to choose not to participate. Scientists have a responsibility to explain the relevance of their work to the people they hope to study, in order for their participation to become what it really is—a collaborative research effort. Only then we can regain some of the trust we have lost.[71]

The documentary registers the efforts of Wells and his colleagues to regain that trust by including representatives of indigenous groups, such as Bluehouse, in their research and by demonstrating their sensitivity to cultural differences. Bluehouse, in fact, has since become a representative of indigenous communities that are participating in the Genographic Project and, in that capacity, attended the public ceremony in Washington, D.C. at which the project was launched. Yet, the IPCB remains unpersuaded; in a press release issued shortly after the announcement of the project, Executive Director Debra Harry called it a 'recurrent nightmare'.[72]

Race as proxy

Journey of Man ends with the familiar anti-racist message about a 'lesson' that 'stands out from all the others. It's a lesson about relationships', Wells observes, against the backdrop of a multiracial group of young adults that resembles (and might be) a photo shoot for a Benetton ad.

> We're all literally African under the skin, brothers and sisters separated by a mere 2000 generations. Old-fashioned concepts of race are not only socially divisive, but scientifically wrong. It's only when we've fully taken this on board that we

---

71 Wells, *The Journey of Man*, 195.
72 Quoted in 'Indigenous peoples oppose National Geographic & IBM genetic research project that seeks indigenous peoples' DNA', IPCB press release, April 13, 2005, available at www.ipcb.org/issues/human_genetics/htmls/geno_pr.html (viewed 22 July 2006).

can say with any conviction that the journey our ancestors launched all those years ago is complete.

Against this message, however, is the familiar language of inevitable extinction that accompanies the affirmation and urgency of the project. Fifteen years ago, Wells explains, from within a Mardi Gras crowd in Rio de Janeiro, depicting globalization and human mixture, scientists lacked the technology to conduct this research and the story could not have been told.

> But, in this era of globalization, isolated populations are being absorbed at an ever increasing rate. It's possible that by the end of the century that [sic] genetic signposts of our journey will have been disbursed around the globe. When this happens, the story will once again become hidden.

Globalization, in this formulation, bleeds into cultural extinction; Wells posits a temporality in which 'indigenous' becomes synonymous with ancestry, and the problems of indigenous communities are cast in terms of cultural preservation rather than racism, poverty and disease. Wells and his colleagues are evidently unaware of how this story perpetuates a particular world-view: how it expresses who and what should be valued and how they should be valued, how resources should be allocated, who will have access to those resources and for what purposes. The story Wells tells in the film is an interpretation; it registers choices about what information will be relevant in determining someone's genealogy, such as the decision to locate the origin of his specific ancestry in Northern Europe. According to the narrative of the film, western civilization has developed ineluctably, and indigenous peoples, in the inevitable and unalterable course of things, become extinct—or pass into the western audience's ancestry. So it is written in the genes. What this account obscures, as I have noted, are the social determinants of development, including the health disparities that evince not the inevitable expression of cultural and biological difference, but the impact of social and economic inequities. Wells's story is written in the language of unacknowledged power as much as genes, and it exemplifies the problem that the organizers of the Howard University symposium underscore as their motivation: that the careless rendition of the genomic story, whether told through medicine or human history, will obscure the social, political and economic sources of outcomes—including health outcomes—and thereby put them beyond investigation. It will, that is, biologize (and naturalize) outcomes that could in fact be addressed and changed.

The sincerity of the scientific refrain that racism has no scientific basis and that scientific racism can be forestalled by explaining the science to the public is apparent. But, as the story of *Journey of Man* makes clear, racism is much more complicated, and much more intricately interwoven in the language, images and stories—the representational conventions—that have

developed with centuries of oppression. The histories—or stories—embedded in our most basic communications are as complex and
difficult to understand as the science. They register (and foster) assumptions
that inevitably become part of genomic information, from the definition of
what constitutes data and the practices through which it is collected to the
narratives through which it is interpreted and applied. Health care
disparities are the result of many factors, some of which can be rectified
by research in genomic medicine. But the narratives that inform the science
and its applications can perpetuate the very inequities they seek to address.

The stories about ancestry that emerge from population genomics can be
incomplete and misleading. Yet they inform many of the assumptions
through which researchers constitute self-identified race and ethnicity as
proxies in the practice of genomic medicine and can therefore influence the
screening, diagnosis and treatment of medical conditions. The language of
urgency permeates the stories and forestalls introspection: if race and
ethnicity can provide useful medical information, it is 'irresponsible' not
to consider them; if indigenous populations are disappearing, we cannot
waste time deliberating about the ethics of DNA sampling. The urgency
obscures the disagreements surrounding the science as well as the lack of
clarity concerning the motivations of the project, and it reinforces the
hierarchy of knowledge. It puts the stories beyond question. It also
conjoins—and recombines—the fields of medical and population genomics;
the medical imperative turns the impending occlusion of the genetic trail
into an apparent loss of valuable medical knowledge.[73] Yet the urgency of
the two fields is in fact at odds: if population intermingling and racial
admixture are becoming the norms, then how useful will self-identified race
and ethnicity be as medical proxies?

Genomic stories have thus reconstituted the biological basis of race as a
central question in scientific research and public discussion at the moment
when, according to population geneticists, cultural and reproductive
intermingling are recombining genomic profiles at unprecedented rates,
hence the threatened 'disappearance' of some genetic markers. Wells calls
DNA a 'global songline' and refers to his account as a 'creation story' of
western science. Throughout *Journey of Man*, he seeks to replace indigenous
accounts with his own migration story, which the loss of 'ancient' markers
threatens to obscure: that is the story he is concerned about losing. Against
the reproductive intermingling that will reshuffle the DNA of all contemporary 'races' and 'populations', *Journey of Man* could be read as a
Euroamerican creation myth written against a perceived threat to the 'racial'
integrity and power of (white) Euroamerica.

---

73 It is interesting to consider how this formulation reproduces the ecological concern
that the disappearance of the rain forest will result in the loss of plants with important
medical properties. 'Indigenous' DNA, in other words, becomes part of the flora and
fauna of the disappearing ecosystem.

That is not, of course, the story Wells and his colleagues intend to tell, but stories, like genes, can be both inherited and mutable. The scientific and public accounts of genomic medicine and human migration risk infusing the genomic creation story with the authority of science and the history of racism. As epistemological technologies, these stories inform the collection and interpretation of data. Reintroducing the biology of race without attending fully to the history of racism is therefore as irresponsible as uncritically dismissing the research. Francis Collins calls for 'more anthropological, sociological and psychological research into how individuals and cultures conceive and internalize concepts of race and ethnicity'.[74] The 'individuals and cultures' under consideration must include the practitioners of western science, and they must consider their cultural investments in their own creation stories.[75] The enquiry needs to begin with an understanding of how the intricate interarticulation of cultural and biological identity is central to health outcomes. Incorporating analyses of these stories—and, specifically, of racism—directly into genomic research is not only ethically and politically correct, it is also good science and medicine.

Priscilla Wald is Professor of English at Duke University and author of *Constituting Americans: Cultural Anxiety and Narrative Form* (Duke University Press 1995) and *Contagion: Cultures, Carriers and the Outbreak Narrative* (forthcoming from Duke). She has also published several essays on genomics, which are part of a book-length manuscript in progress.

74 Collins, 'What we do and don't know about "race," "ethnicity," genetics and health at the dawn of the genome era', S14.
75 Collins follows this recommendation with another that calls for researchers to 'assess how the scientific community uses the concepts of race and ethnicity and attempt to remedy situations in which the use of such concepts is misleading or counterproductive' (ibid., S15). As I have been arguing throughout this essay, such an examination of vocabulary and other representational practices is crucial, but genomic researchers need to understand the problem as more than one of vocabulary and miscommunication. Cultural assumptions and biases are embedded in and perpetuated by the tools of communication, and western societies must be understood as 'cultures' with their own sets of beliefs and practices. The recent move in anthropology that has made it increasingly acceptable to do fieldwork in one's own culture marks an important turn; the laboratories of researchers, in fact, have increasingly become sites for anthropological fieldwork.

Alcohol and the Jews (again), race and medicine (again): on race and medicine in historical perspective

SANDER L. GILMAN

ABSTRACT   The question of why or whether Jews have a resistance to alcoholism is now the subject of genetic research. Parallel to investigations into such perceived resistance in other groups (such as 'Asians'), the recent work makes global claims that can be shown to have very specific social and historical origins. The accusation that the Jews abused alcohol was rebutted in the eighteenth century as Jews entered into the German-speaking public sphere. The key to such access was adherence to rules of 'decorum', and the public consumption of alcohol was central to this project.

With the first patent being granted on 15 October 2002 for a medication (BiDil) deemed to be most effective for a specific 'race', African Americans, for a specific form of heart failure, the ongoing debate about the effect of the older category of 'race' has been revitalized.[1] What role should race play in the discussion of the genetic make-up of populations today? The new genetics seems to make 'race' a category that is useful if not necessary, as the *New York Times* noted recently: 'Race-based prescribing makes sense only as a temporary measure.'[2] Should one think about 'race' as a transitional category that is of some use while we continue to explore the actual genetic make-up of and relationships in populations? Or is such a transitional solution poisoning the actual research and practice? Given the recent breakthrough in mapping genetic variation with potential attention to pathologies (the International HapMap project) among peoples across wide geographic areas (China, Japan, Nigeria and the United States), the idea that

---

1 BiDil is a combination of two drugs, hydralazine and isosorbide dinitrate (H/I). These drugs are vasodilators: they dilate blood vessels in order to diminish the stress on the heart as it pumps blood. The study that determined this was Peter Carson, S. Ziesche, G. Johnson, J. N. Cohn, 'Racial differences in response to therapy for heart failure: analysis of the vasodilator-heart failure trials', *Journal of Cardiac Failure*, vol. 5, 1999, 178–87. See R. Kittles and C. Royal, 'The genetics of African Americans: implications for disease gene mapping and identity', in Alan H. Goodman, Deborah Heath and M. Susan Lindee (eds), *Genetic Nature/Culture: Anthropology and Science beyond the Two-Culture Divide* (Berkeley: University of California Press 2003), 219–33.
2 'Toward the first racial medicine', *New York Times*, 13 November 2004.

'race' is helpful in the understanding and treatment of common disorders such as heart disease, cancer and diabetes is truly suspect.[3] Charles Rotimi, a professor in the College of Medicine at Howard University, one of the universities that sponsors the mapping project, said that the results supported scientists' understanding of genetic variation as continuous across populations, not sharply divided into racial categories.[4]

The irony is that when in November 2005 a letter appeared in *Nature Genetics* online that provided some further data on the BiDil claim of effectiveness its authors wrote of 'ethnicity-specific risk of myocardial infarction'.[5] By 2005, not 'race' but 'ethnicity' seemed to be the key to a higher rate of heart disease among African Americans. Yet the label of 'ethnicity' is an odd one. The authors, from Iceland and the United States, argued that there seemed to be a 'three-fold risk' among 'African Americans' (unhyphenated) of heart attacks, as 27 per cent of 'European Americans' carried the gene variants that might moderate the 'risk of myocardial infarction'. But what do the unhyphenated labels reflecting 'ethnicity' mean in this context? They have nothing to do with 'ethnicity' as a means by which an individual understands being in a cohort. The German sociologist Max Weber (1864–1920) defined 'ethnicity' as 'the belief in group affinity', which, 'regardless of whether it has any objective foundation, can have important consequences especially for the formation of a political community'.[6]

But this belief in one's own ethnicity is belied by the authors of this letter who 'corrected for potentially misclassified individuals by excluding from the study self-reported African Americans with < 20% African genetic ancestry ...' With this pattern of exclusion, they claimed an objective (genetic) basis for 'ethnicity'. Here the category is not truly 'ethnicity' but it is also not 'race'. What the study relied on were the statistics of genetic frequency. The claim was that the Icelandic and the Nigerian (Yoruba) HapMap provided indices of group genetic identity based on the absence or presence of the genetic marker for resistance to heart attacks. This claim was muddled by the authors' use of 'European American' as a genetic category. It was included one assumes because of the assumption, made evident in a press conference by one of the authors, that 'the more active version of this

3 The International HapMap Consortium, 'A haplotype map of the human genome', *Nature*, vol. 437, October 2005, 1299–320.

4 See Lila Guterman, 'Scientists release map of human genetic variation that may help treat common diseases', *Chronicle of Higher Education* (online only), 27 October 2005.

5 Anna Helgadottir, Andrei Manolescu, Agnar Helgason, Gudmar Thorleifsson *et al.*, 'A variant of the gene encoding leukotriene A4 hydrolase confers ethnicity-specific risk of myocardial infarction', *Nature Genetics* (online), 10 November 2005 (print publication in vol. 38, no. 1, January 2006).

6 Max Weber, 'Ethnic groups (1922)', in Werner Sollors (ed.), *Theories of Ethnicity: A Classical Reader* (New York: New York University Press 1996), 56. See also Werner Sollors (ed.), *The Invention of Ethnicity* (New York: Oxford University Press 1988).

gene might have risen to prominence in Europeans and Asians because it conferred extra protection against infectious diseases'.[7] Such 'just so stories' beg the obvious questions why Africans (seen here as a homogeneous category even though the group utilized was a specific one, the Yoruba) did not need such protection, and whether this makes them a 'sickly race', to use the nineteenth-century term. What the study does seem to show is that certain genetic groups may have a statistical resistance to certain types of inflammation that may be correlated to heart attacks. It certainly does not make much of an argument for 'ethnicity' as a category of analysis. The anxiety about the label 'race' evident in the study is perhaps as interesting as the claims for the identification of risk among a population that is (self-)defined by the category of 'race'. Is the initial response to risk a desire to 'map' 'African Americans' to exclude from that 'ethnic' community those who are 'too white'? Is this not a 'racial' category?

Race presents both epidemiological and historical problems for the society in which it is raised as well as for medical research and practice. Clearly, after the Holocaust, we are shy about using 'race' as a category, even when we seem to be correcting imbalances, such as those in medical testing that ignore women and minorities.[8] 'Ethnicity' seems an odd means of avoiding the associations of 'race'. The rebirth of 'race' in the twenty-first century has changed the very contours of its meaning. 'Race' has thus expanded to cover a wide range of meanings from common ancestry to shared history to geographic spaces. While its origin, as much of the recent literature illustrates, is clearly biological, over the past decades it has come to be used interchangeably with 'ethnicity', 'ancestry', 'culture', 'colour', 'national origin' and even 'religion'.[9] But who defines 'race'? The self-defined group, the government, the research funder, the researcher? What does one do with what are deemed 'race-specific' diseases, such as 'Jewish genetic diseases', that are so defined because they are often concentrated in a group but are also found beyond the group? Are we comfortable designating 'Jews' or 'African Americans' as 'races' given their genetic diversity? One must note that professional associations, such as the American Anthropological Association, rejected, as late as 1998, the use of 'race' as a 'scientific' category as it involved the creation of a hierarchy that would 'assign some

---

7 Nicholas Wade, 'Gene find links race, heart risk', *Atlanta Journal-Constitution*, 11 November 2005, A1, A9 (this article was entitled 'Genetic find stirs debate on race-based medicine' when it was published that same day in the *New York Times*). One large component of the study was undertaken in Atlanta at Emory University.

8 Jacqueline Stevens, 'Racial meanings and scientific methods: changing policies for NIH-sponsored publications reporting human variation', *Journal of Health Politics, Policy and Law*, vol. 28, 2003, 1033–88.

9 There is a huge literature on the concept of 'race', from John S. Haller, *Outcasts from Evolution: Scientific Attitudes of Racial Inferiority, 1859–1900* (Urbana: University of Illinois Press 1971) to George Stocking, 'The turn-of-the-century concept of race', *Modernism/Modernity*, vol. 1, no. 1, 1994, 4–16, and beyond.

groups to perpetual low status, while others were permitted access to privilege, power, and wealth'.[10]

Yet medicine seems comfortable for political reasons to reintroduce 'race' as 'a real, natural phenomenon', a phrase used by the American Anthropological Association in 1997 in its rejection of the use of 'race' for being neither 'real' nor 'natural'.[11] The politics, at least in the United States, are 'liberal' in their rhetoric.[12] The demand is to include diversity in the testing of all pharmaceuticals. Diversity means the inclusion of women and 'minorities', the latter defined by the prevailing categories used in the most recent census. It thus includes self-defined ethnic categories, such as 'African American', but also constructed composite categories, such as 'Asian American'. The recent use of 'ethnicity' as an alternative label for 'race' is claimed to be just as 'real' and 'natural'. Behind every nuanced recycling of the concept of 'race' as something else lurks the anthropological origin of the term with its claims of biological objectivity. Given that anthropological categories of 'race' dominated nineteenth-century medicine, this present disjuncture is of importance.[13] Accordingly, original and clearly groundbreaking work on population and individual genetics remains in thrall to older 'racial' categories, which deform and undermine the implication of its science.

Alcoholism and 'Jewish' genes

One category that has been 'medicalized' in the very recent past in terms of race is alcoholism. Recently there has been an attempt to look for a genetic basis both for this disease and for its absence. In this case, it is as if the norm is the disease. Thus, there is a commonplace that Jews do not drink to excess. Most recently, John Efron in his magisterial *Medicine and the German Jews* has argued for the genetic hypothesis: Jews are genetically not predisposed to alcoholism.[14] Efron evokes the medical model that sees alcoholism as inherited, which has been dominant over the past fifty years. It was

---

10 American Anthropological Association, 'Statement on "race"', 17 May 1998, available at www.aaanet.org/stmts/racepp.htm (viewed 29 June 2006).
11 American Anthropological Association, 'Response to OMB Directive 15: race and ethnic standards for federal statistics and administrative reporting', September 1997, available at www.aaanet.org/gvt/ombdraft.htm (viewed 29 June 2006). The Association suggested the substitution of 'ethnicity' or 'ethnic group'.
12 Esteban González Burchard, Elad Ziv, Natasha Coyle, Scarlett Lin Gomez, Hua Tang, Andrew J. Karter, Joanna L. Mountain, Eliseo J. Pérez-Stable, Dean Sheppard and Neil Risch, 'The importance of race and ethnic background in biomedical research and clinical practice', *New England Journal of Medicine*, vol. 348, no. 12, March 2003, 1170–5.
13 Guido Barbujani, 'Human races: classifying people vs. understanding diversity', *Current Genomics*, vol. 6, no. 4, 2005, 215–26.
14 John Efron, *Medicine and the German Jews: A History* (New Haven: Yale University Press 2001), 108–17.

introduced after the Second World War as a calculated attempt to replace the moral model positing a lack of will with a model of collective predisposition.[15] Such a model, it was assumed, freed individuals who were 'alcoholics' from the stigma of individual responsibility for their 'addiction'. It was a genetic fault or mutation in the collective (race) that was at the heart of the matter.

The high (or low) point of this came in 2001 when the gene for the resistance to alcoholism in 'Jews' was supposedly discovered.[16] In a paper published that year a group of researchers based in San Diego argued that they had

> evaluated 84 Ashkenazic Jewish American college students to determine the prevalence of the ADH2*2 allele (0.31). Carriers of ADH2*2 reported significantly fewer drinking days per month. ADH2*2, however, was not related to alcohol use disorders, alcohol-induced flushing and associated symptoms, number of binge drinking episodes in the past 90 days, maximum number of drinks ever consumed, or self-reported levels of response to alcohol. Results suggest that Ashkenazic Jewish Americans with ADH2*2 alleles drink less frequently, which might contribute, in part, to the overall lower rates of alcoholism in this population.[17]

In other words, among Jewish college students of 'Ashkenazic' descent, alcoholism is less apparent. But what does this actually mean? The authors understand the dangers of the claims and dismiss them.

> Other limitations of this study included the use of self-report data, which may have produced increased variability. Study measures, however, were shown to have good reliability and validity and ADH2 gene status was not known at the time of data collection. Moreover, the sample consisted only of Ashkenazic college

15 Mariana Valverde, *Diseases of the Will: Alcohol and the Dilemmas of Freedom* (Cambridge: Cambridge University Press 1998), esp. 'The Jews vs. the Irish', 115–19. This debate is presented in much greater detail in Charles R. Snyder, *Alcohol and the Jews: A Cultural Study of Drinking and Sobriety* (Carbondale: Southern Illinois University Press 1978). See also Louis Lieberman, 'Jewish alcoholism and the disease concept', *Journal of Psychology and Judaism*, vol. 11, 1987, 165–80; K. C. M. Loewenthal, *Alcohol and Suicide Related Ideas and Behaviour among Jews and Protestants* (London: Economic and Social Research Council 2002); and Kate M. Loewenthal, Michelle Lee, Andrew K. Macleod, Susan Cook and Vivienne Goldblatt, 'Drowning your sorrows? Attitudes towards alcohol in U.K. Jews and Protestants: a thematic analysis', *International Journal of Social Psychiatry*, vol. 49, September 2003, 204–15.
16 Shoshana H. Shea, Tamara L. Wall, Lucinda G. Carr and Ting-kai Li, 'ADH2 and alcohol-related phenotypes in Ashkenazic Jewish American college students', *Behavior Genetics*, vol. 31, no. 2, March 2001, 231–9.
17 Ibid., 231. An allele is any of two or more alternative forms of a gene that occupy the same locus on a chromosome.

students, so the findings may not generalize to all Jewish Americans, such as Sephardic Jews or older populations.[18]

But it is not just alcohol use that is self-reported; even the category of 'Ashkenazic college students' is a self-reported one. What did this mean in the United States in 2001, looking at the fourth or fifth generation of Americans from Central and Eastern Europe? The assumption is that these cadres continued to follow the romanticized marriage practices of Eastern Europe, a fact that the anxiety about intermarriage over the past forty years in the United States seems to obviate. The 'Jews' in the study respond similarly to the 'Asians':

> A variety of genetically influenced alcohol-related phenotypes relate to risk for alcohol dependence. In Asians, variation in the alcohol dehydrogenase (ADH2*2) gene relates to alcohol dependence, alcohol consumption, and reported alcohol-related symptoms, even after controlling for variation in the aldehyde dehydrogenase (ALDH2*2) gene. The association of ADH2*2 polymorphisms with alcohol-related behavior, however, has not been well characterized in non Asians.[19]

But of course 'Asian' is a very American category, lumping diverse cultures, histories and geographies into a handy group for census purposes. Likewise, 'the Ashkenazic Jews' are a construction of often contradictory meanings. Both are attempts to create a genetic homogeneity out of diverse and ever changing populations. The authors are, of course, inchoate in their attempt to define the categories of 'Asians' and 'Jews'. Based on these claims further genes for alcohol resistance were found.

> 'We know that alcoholism is hereditary,' said Cindy L. Ehlers, associate professor of neuropharmacology at the Scripps Research Institute and lead author of a later study that claimed to document this genetic resistance to alcoholism by looking more broadly beyond the 'Jews and Asians' in 2002. 'But we only have very limited information on what is inherited, and almost no information on what genes might be involved except in the case of alcohol metabolizing enzymes.'[20]

The gene this group discovered is on the ADH2*3 site. Commentary on this finding notes that a related genetic pattern seems to be the reason for the absence of alcoholism among 'Jews':

18 Ibid., 237.
19 Ibid., 236.
20 David A. Gilder, Tamara L. Wall and Cindy L. Ehlers, 'Psychiatric diagnoses among mission Indian children with and without a parental history of alcohol dependence', *Journal of Studies on Alcohol*, vol. 63, January 2002, 18–23.

'We would predict that the frequency of ADH2*3 will be lower in the alcoholics than in the non-alcoholics,' David W. Crabb, professor of medicine, biochemistry and molecular biology, and chair of the Department of Medicine at Indiana University Medical Center observed. 'Similar findings have been obtained with individuals with another high-activity ADH allele, ADH2*2, that is found in Asians and Jews.'[21]

You can observe how a small group of 'Ashkenazic Jewish' college students has become the 'Jews'. The problem with all of these findings is that they make assumptions about the constitution of 'populations' from the genetic make-up of individuals or families. They then extrapolate a general genetic key for the resistance to alcoholism from that small sample, as if 'resistance' were a behavioural reflex of that gene.[22]

The idea that 'my genes made me do it (or not do it)' remains the mantra for understanding alcoholism as an addiction. I (among many others) have not been convinced that alcoholism fulfils the necessary requirements to be understood as a disease, or, indeed, that dependence on alcohol has a single cause, certainly not a solely genetic one. But to reverse the argument and claim that there is a protective genetic component that shields a group such as the 'Jews' is a rather odd extension of the medical argument explaining resistance. This was a commonplace of nineteenth-century medicine, when the question was asked in 1854, for example, 'to what agent or agents are the Jews indebted for their reported exemption from cholera?'[23] Such questions revealed themselves even at the time to be specious, as it turned out that Jews developed cholera just as frequently as anyone else.[24] While suspicion fell on 'their intermarriage, the race being pure', as having 'some influence in excluding extraneous sources of hereditary disease', the social context was also assumed.[25] What British physicians had long known was that the Jews, then defined as members of an institution, the synagogue, quickly banded together to provide medical care for their co-religionists, a model that was advocated for all groups in London.[26] It is access to treatment and

---

21 'Researchers find gene mutation that protects against addiction', *Pain and Central Nervous System Week*, 7 January 2002, 2.
22 This argument was made as early as 1990 by Troy Duster in *Backdoor to Eugenics* (New York: Routledge 1990), 3–20, and by him (with Pilar Ossorio) in 'Race and genetics: controversies in biomedical, behavioral, and forensic sciences', *American Psychologist*, vol. 60, January 2005, 115–28.
23 J. H. Tucker, 'To what agent or agents are the Jews indebted for their reported exemption from cholera', *The Lancet*, vol. 64, 30 December 1854, 552.
24 Edward Greenhow, 'Alleged exemption of Jews from cholera', *The Lancet*, vol. 65, 13 January 1855, 50; answered by J. H. Tucker, 'Alleged exemption of the Jews from cholera', *The Lancet*, vol. 65, 27 January 1855, 110.
25 'The health of Jews', *The Lancet*, vol. 105, 3 April 1875, 484.
26 Thomas Lloyd, 'Prompt medical attendance on the poor', *The Lancet*, vol. 29, 16 December 1837, 456.

preventative measures, and a question of reporting the incidence of disease, that create the illusion of immunity.

Today the question of the genetic component of behavioural or social 'ills' has reappeared with a vengeance. Contemporary medicine has even reintroduced the concept of 'race' (which had never truly vanished) because of the politics of medical multiculturalism. The entire question of whether the 'Jews' or the 'Irish' or the 'Native Americans' are appropriate designations for genetic variation or even comprehensible descriptors of statistical populations is again debated, but almost always with regard to the inclusion of a 'race' as the site of illness, rarely with regard to its exclusion. The concomitant question of whether behaviour is always genetically determined seems to be a central part of this new fascination with race. Yet, as nineteenth-century physicians well knew, once the concept of 'race' is used in medicine it can be used to 'explain' virtually anything.[27]

Even in studies in which a non-genetic explanation for the Jews' relationship to alcohol is sought, the result is completely determined by how the term 'Jews' is used as a descriptor. Thus, one recent study in the United Kingdom on Jews, alcohol and depression used self-reporting to define the 'Jews' and discovered that 'Jews had less favourable beliefs about alcohol and drank less than Protestants'.[28] At the same time, a study in Israel found that 'Arabs tend to favor restrictive attitudes toward alcohol control measures in comparison with Jews'.[29] Indeed, if you move from 'Jew' to 'Israeli' (but still defined as 'Jewish'), the concern arises that 'a worrisome prevalence of non-ritual alcohol use among Israelis [has] reinforced the position that the phenomenon of drinking is liable to develop into an important social and public health problem in the State of Israel'.[30] The 'cure' for this problem is seen as rooted in individual character traits, not in any type of group response.[31] Clearly, these are very different ideas of who is a 'Jew'. Indeed, a recent survey of the literature on Jews and drinking

27 For a case study, see John S. Haller, 'The Negro and the southern physician: a study of medical and racial attitudes, 1800–1860', *Medical History*, vol. 16, no. 3, 1972, 238–53.
28 Kate M. Loewenthal, Andrew K. MacLeod, Susan Cook, Michelle Lee and Vivienne Goldblatt, 'Beliefs about alcohol among UK Jews and Protestants: do they fit the alcohol-depression hypothesis?', *Social Psychiatry and Psychiatric Epidemiology*, vol. 38, no. 3, March 2003, 122–7.
29 Shoshana Weiss, 'Attitudes of Israeli Jewish and Arab high school students toward alcohol control measures', *Journal of Drug Education*, vol. 29, no. 1, 1999, 41–52.
30 Haviva Bar, Pnina Eldar and Shoshana Weiss, 'Alcohol drinking habits and attitudes of the adult Jewish population in Israel 1987', *Drug and Alcohol Dependence*, vol. 23, no. 3, June 1989, 237–45.
31 Rachel Lev-Wiesel, 'The right stuff: key personality characteristics that indicate success in overcoming addiction in Israel', in Richard Isralowitz, Mohammed Afifi and Richard Rawson (eds), *Drug Problems: Cross-Cultural Policy and Program Development* (Westport, CT and London: Auburn House 2002), 233–42.

dismissed the claim of a Jewish (no matter how defined) immunity to alcoholism in general as an unfounded assumption.[32]

The long story of Jews and alcohol

The debate today about Jews and alcohol seems to be one about the claim for a genetic immunity of the Jews to alcoholism. That there seems to be little consensus about how to define either 'Jews' or 'alcoholism' makes this claim difficult to accept. There may well be some individuals for whom a set of genetic markers (combined with a complex set of triggering experiences) predisposes them to a greater risk of becoming (or not becoming) addicted to alcohol. But the entire discussion about a 'Jewish' immunity to alcoholism assumes that there has always been a public awareness of Jewish 'moderation'. The reality is that this assumption (and the social practice that it may or may not lead to) is part of the process of modernization that includes the integration of Jews into western social habits and mores.[33] Rhetoric about decorum used (and uses) public drunkenness as a marker of unacceptable social behaviour. Indeed, it is 'public drunkenness' that defines alcohol abuse in the public mind from the Enlightenment to the Women's Christian Temperance Union pledge not to drink alcohol adopted in 1894 and beyond. What I am interested in is the establishment of the assumption that an excess of alcohol use leads to a lack of decorum and how that assumption becomes a part of the modern world of Jews in German-speaking lands. Jews had to adopt within their religious practice the same degree of public decorum as was imagined to exist among their Protestant neighbours. This is not a claim about whether Jews were or were not prone to alcohol abuse before or after the Enlightenment; it is merely a claim about public attitudes towards Jews and alcohol from the eighteenth century to the present. I do not wish to be reductive in this argument and thus parallel the monocausal explanation of contemporary genetics for the 'fact' of Jewish resistance to alcoholism. What I argue is that being 'Jewish' and being 'decorous' become so entwined by the 1790s that there is no way of easily untangling them, even to the point of

---

32 Steven L. Berg, *Jewish Alcoholism and Drug Addiction: An Annotated Bibliography* (Westport, CT: Greenwood Press 1993).

33 In general, see the more recent works by David Sorkin, *The Berlin Haskalah and German Religious Thought: Orphans of Knowledge* (London: Vallentine Mitchell 2000); Michael A. Meyer, *Judaism within Modernity: Essays on Jewish History and Religion* (Detroit: Wayne State University Press 2001); Jonathan M. Hess, *Germans, Jews and the Claims of Modernity* (New Haven, CT and London: Yale University Press 2002); Arno Herzig, Hans Otto Horch and Robert Jütte (eds), *Judentum und Aufklärung: jüdisches Selbstverständnis in der bürgerlichen Öffentlichkeit* (Göttingen: Vandenhoeck and Ruprecht 2002); Jeremy Asher Dauber, *Antonio's Devils: Writers of the Jewish Enlightenment and the Birth of Modern Hebrew and Yiddish Literature* (Stanford, CA: Stanford University Press 2004).

examining the internalization of such images in the construction of modern Jewish identity.

If one can trace this to a single point of origin it is to the public letter that Moses Mendelssohn wrote to the Swiss preacher Johann Caspar Lavater in 1769 in which he countered Lavater's demand that he either refute the truths of Christianity or convert. Mendelssohn's careful answer stresses the need for a sense of decorum in public debate, which cannot exist under such demands. His enlightened friends, such as Gotthold Ephraim Lessing, seemed to agree, since Lessing's 'Nathan the Wise' (who captures Lessing's image of Mendelssohn) is a model of public decorousness. Indeed, Mendelssohn's defence of Judaism in his *Jerusalem* (1783) does not make it into a 'rational' religion, as some later claimed, but into a decorous one.

In April 1790 Paul Jakob Bruns (1743–1814), in an essay in the *Berlinische Monatsschrift*, addressed the question of whether the Jews should abandon the festival of Purim, the holiday celebrating the rescue of the Persian Jews by Esther from the machinations of Haman.[34] Bruns was one of the most noted biblical scholars of his day and, at the time he wrote this essay, was a historian, theologian, professor of Oriental literature and librarian of the University at Helmstädt. After that university was closed in 1810 he taught for over three decades at Halle. In his 1790 essay Bruns deplores the very act that rescues the Jews of Persia; the joy expressed by the Jews in the routing and destruction of their enemies is unseemly, as the act does not reflect 'great deeds or persons that showed bravery and power for the improvement of their fatherland'.[35] Rather, the Jews appear to be weak and whiney, to mourn their own fate and to wear that mourning before anything occurs, and then to kill innocent people in vengeance. Indeed, Esther's very act is not a great 'expression of the soul' but rather done grudgingly, showing the inherently weak character of the Jews. At the centre of this tale, Bruns writes, is the desire for vengeance on the part of the Jews against their oppressors.[36] He notes that the Jews of his day imagine their treatment by the Christians being revenged if only through the memory of their defeat of the Persians.

---

34 Paul Jakob Bruns, 'Vorschlag an die Juden, das Purimfest abzuschaffen', *Berlinische Monatsschrift*, April 1790, 377–80. Bruns was a polymath but was best known in his time as the author of *Neue systematische Erdbeschreibung von Africa* (Nuremberg: Schneider und Weigel 1799) and *Beiträge zur kritischen Bearbeitung unbenutzter alter Handschriften, Drucke und Urkunden*, 3 vols (Braunschweig: Reichard 1802–3). He also edited *Martin Luthers ungedruckte Predigten* (Helmstädt: Fleckeisen 1796).

35 Bruns, 'Vorschlag an die Juden', 378. Translations from the German, unless otherwise stated, are by the author.

36 What Bruns does not do is to evoke the older image of the hanging of Haman as a parody of the Crucifixion. This image may well be part of the mediaeval rhetoric associated with the blood libel. See Cecil Roth, 'The feast of Purim and the origins of the blood accusation', *Speculum*, vol. 8, no. 4, October 1933, 520–6 and Gerd Mentgen, 'Über den Ursprung der Ritualmordfabel', *Aschkenas*, vol. 4, 1994, 405–16.

Bruns's argument centres on the character of the Jews as reflected in the story of Purim and the application of that tale to the world of eighteenth-century Jewry. He acknowledges that the Jews are in the midst of reform and suggests that they should strongly look at the celebration of Purim as it reveals the innate incompatibility of Jewish ritual with German sensibility. His reference is to the model evoked in Christian Wilhelm von Dohm's plan for the 'civic improvement of the Jews': Jews must transform themselves in order to become citizens of the state. They must reject or reform practices that are understood as inimical to that goal. This is very much in contrast to the views of other contemporaries, such as the liberal educational reformer Wilhelm von Humboldt, who, following John Locke, saw an inherent right to citizenship no matter what one's religious practices. Mendelssohn and most Jewish followers of the Enlightenment agreed with Dohm's position. Bruns cites the disorder among children in the synagogue who drown out the name of Haman with wooden clappers as a sign of the lack of proper decorum. Central to his argument is the 'exaggeration of gluttony (*fressen*) and drunkenness (*saufen*)' that accompanies the holiday.[37] These terms themselves, and their link with the Purim 'comedies' that are played as part of the celebration, point to the notion that Jews are lacking in public decorum. Indeed, 'Christians have disgust and disrespect for the entire nation [of the Jews]', and even 'the philosophers among the Jews' are exasperated by these extravagances.[38] Bruns's source, if he has one that is more precise than the word-of-mouth 'common wisdom' of his time, may well have been texts such as Johann Jakob Schudt's early eighteenth-century accounts of Jewish holidays and beliefs.[39] Schudt begins his account of Purim with a condemnation of the 'haughtiness and insolence' of the Jews of the time who spend their time with 'gaming, gluttony (*fressen*) and inebriation (*saufen*)'. The Jews of Frankfurt, for example, 'riot, eat and drink and undertake all sorts of amusements'.[40] They attend Purim plays that are little better than 'shit' (*Mist*). This is a blanket condemnation of the festivities that are seen as a form of extravagance violating the accepted order. Bruns's suggestion is simply to stop celebrating the holiday. It is a secular celebration, not prescribed by the Mosaic law. He stresses this point, which was the rationale for the continuance of many Jewish rituals (including circumcision) among Enlightenment Jews. He concludes with a simple threat: if the Jews do not stop such celebrations, the state authorities will. Order must prevail. No excess within ritual can be tolerated as it under-mines the very nature of the state by mocking it as being no more in control of the Jews than were the Persians.

37 Bruns, 'Vorschlag an die Juden', 380.
38 Ibid.
39 Johann Jakob Schudt, *Jüdische Merckwürdigkeiten*, 4 vols (Frankfurt and Leipzig 1714), vol. 2, sec. 6, ch. 35, 308–16.
40 Ibid., 308, 314.

David Friedländer (1750–1834), perhaps the most radical thinker among the Jewish Enlightenment figures of his time, counters Bruns's suggestion almost immediately.[41] In a powerful polemic, he takes on Bruns's arguments point by point, always circling back to the question of decorum. He begins by asking how one can observe the mot in one's neighbour's eye while ignoring the beam in one's own. 'Helpful' criticism of the Jews and their rituals in the light of Dohm's earlier position now seems to take on a negative, destructive tone in which the 'narration of the religious prejudices of strange followers of other religions' reflects a pleasure at their 'comic' nature.[42] At least, the argument seems to go, we Christians are not so silly as to do such things. Friedländer stresses early in his presentation the difference in the development of *Bildung* (here 'acculturation') among the Jews of Prussia, Austria, France and Poland, noting that most of the 'Jews' whom Bruns addresses could not even read his essay.[43] Those who could read it had already fulfilled his moral expectations. The Jews of Prussia, among whom Friedländer counts himself, are the most sensitive to such views and had already modified their ritual practice, 'even though there may be many Jewish children in Prussia who use the clapper at Purim and many adults who drink to excess (*berauschet*) on this day'.[44] Given Friedländer's desire to strip Jewish practice of most ritual, as his suggestions for the radical reform of the Kassel Jewish community a decade later show, this state of affairs still needed to be tended to.

Friedländer stresses, in accord with Bruns, that the true reward for such alterations in religious practice is the improvement of the entire community rather than the improvement of the individual. Yet he argues that such charges as made by Bruns do not necessarily lead to the acquisition of *Bildung* among the Jews but rather reflect the entrenched, pre-Enlightenment views of the nature of the Jewish character: that is, the Jews were 'accused of violating their oaths, of being too attached to Palestine, or being pygmy-like in their stature, or having the advantage of not dueling on the Sabbath'.[45] These accusations, then, are simply re-enforcing stereotypes that do not need re-enforcing, but countering.

Friedländer puts Bruns's views on Purim into this category. He stresses that Bruns's reading of the moral implications of the tale of Esther is simply

---

41 [David Friedländer], 'Freimüthige Gedanken eines Juden über den Vorschlag an die Juden, das Purimfest abzuschaffen', *Berlinische Monatsschrift*, 1790, 563–77. See Steven M. Lowenstein, *The Jewishness of David Friedländer and the Crisis of Berlin Jewry*, Braun Lectures in the History of the Jews in Prussia, 3 (Ramat-Gan: Bar-Ilan University Press 1994).
42 [Friedländer], 'Freimüthige Gedanken eines Juden', 563.
43 Ibid., 565.
44 Ibid., 566.
45 Ibid., 568.

wrong. The bloodthirstiness of the Jews, the nasty, whining, cringing nature of their character, is simply, according to Friedländer, not to be found in the Book of Esther (*Megillah*). To this end, Friedländer's quotes from Luther's translation of the Book of Esther,[46] as well as from contemporary Protestant readings of it by theologians such as Johann Gottfried Eichhorn, the founder of the 'Higher Criticism' of the 'Old' Testament.[47] He counters that the celebration of Purim is a necessary part of the ritual practices of the Jews as it is not detrimental to the 'common man'.[48] He can work on the feast day and need only spend an extra hour in the evening listening to the text of the Book of Esther being read aloud in synagogue. Bruns's central point, that this text is understood not as a historical record of the rescue of the Jews of Persia but as a desired overpowering of the Christian states in which they now live, is dismissed by Friedländer in a most remarkable manner. He argues that he is not entirely in favour of retaining the misuse of the festival of Purim, especially the excess of drinking and eating (*Schwelgen*). For what the Jews in the synagogues think about when they hear the Book of Esther read is neither the overcoming of Haman nor the possible application of such a *coup d'état* to contemporary states but the 'feast (*Schmauß*) that awaits them and that remedies the fast day that had occurred; he stamps with his feet when he hears the name of Haman, because his fathers had done so ...'.[49] In Prussia, such 'immoralities were being lost and the rough edges [of the Jews] smoothed'.[50]

> Even if in Berlin the clapper has not completely disappeared, the Purim comedies, the drunkenness, and other excesses of an excessive happiness ... either never existed or have been long abandoned. At least I have ... neither seen nor heard about such things.[51]

Indeed, the tradition of the lack of decorum and the interruption of the somber ritual of prayer in connection with Purim come to be seen as a hallmark of the ritual practices of the mediaeval German-Jewish world by reformers such as Leopold Zunz.[52] Friedländer charges his readers to abandon the generalities about the Jews and their lack of decorum and the threat that such a lack poses for the society in which they live. It is the duty of the 'stronger', he notes, 'to extend an arm to the weaker' and 'say "let us be friends"'.[53] This is not achieved by Bruns's exaggerated carping demands

46 Ibid., 569.
47 Ibid., 571.
48 Ibid., 573.
49 Ibid., 575.
50 Ibid.
51 Ibid., 576.
52 Leopold Zunz, *Die Ritus des synagogalen Gottesdienstes, geschichtlich entwickelt*, 2 vols (Berlin: J. Springer 1855–9), ii.69.
53 [Friedländer], 'Freimüthige Gedanken eines Juden', 576.

that the Jews alter their religious practices.[54] Indeed, these only exacerbate hatred of the Jews by stressing the corrupt nature of the manner by which they worship and act.

Such a position is very much in line with the general tenor of the time in terms of decorum. Two years earlier, in 1788, Adolf Freiherr von Knigge published his guide to social interaction, without doubt the single most important statement of the Enlightenment concept of decorum.[55] He warns (and I quote a contemporary British translation) that 'nothing can be more disgusting to a sensible man, than the sight of a rational being depriving himself of the use of his intellects by too copious draughts of that exhilarating beverage'.[56] The sober Enlightened man has the duty

> not to indulge them in their excesses, how pleasing so ever the shape maybe in which they appear, but to shew as far as prudence permits that you have an unconquerable aversion against them, and to be particularly careful never to join in smutty discourses.[57]

The description would fit Bruns's and other earlier descriptions of the Jews at Purim, with the excess of alcohol and the lewd Purim plays. But Knigge's discussion of social intercourse with the Jews focused obsessively on Jews and money, Jews and trade, Jews and haggling.[58]

This is typical of the Enlightenment. Both Montesquieu in *De l'esprit des lois* (1748) and David Hume in his essay 'Of National Characters' (1748) agree with Knigge about the public nature of the Jews.[59] Each, however, has his own explanation: Montesquieu believes that it rests on the 'nature' of the Jew; Hume, on their political context. Knigge's image of the Jew is an Enlightenment one that perpetuates in different rhetorical guise the notion of an essential Jewish sensibility. But in his third edition of 1794 Knigge notes that he is not speaking about those 'who have (perhaps not for their own happiness) transformed themselves to follow the morals of Christians'. That is, he is not speaking of those Jews who have begun to transform themselves

---

54 Bruns's rhetoric seems to have a history among 'modern' theologians. See the Amsterdam theologian Philippe (Philipp) van (de) Limborch, *De veritate religionis Christianae, amica collatio cum erudito Judaeo* (Gouda: Apud Justum ab Hoeve 1687), a screed against all forms of Jewish ritual practice as defended by Uriel Acosta. It was to Limborch that John Locke addressed his famed 'Letter on Toleration' (1685). This was his answer.

55 Adolf Freiherr von Knigge, *Ueber den Umgang mit Menschen*, 3rd edn, 3 vols (Frankfurt and Leipzig 1794).

56 Adolf Freiherr von Knigge, *Practical Philosophy of Social Life*, trans. from the German by Peter Will, 2 vols (London: T. Cadell 1796), ii.106.

57 Ibid., i.139.

58 Knigge, *Ueber den Umgang mit Menschen*, iii.115–20 (117). See also Ruth Klüger, *Knigges 'Umgang mit Menschen'* (Göttingen: Wallstein 1996), 15–16.

59 See Nathan Rotenstreich, *The Recurring Pattern. Studies in Anti-Judaism in Modern Thought* (London: Weidenfeld and Nicolson 1963), 23–47 (on Kant).

into 'Germans'. For these Jews, Knigge complains, Christian sins and foolishness replace the simplicity and moral rigour of their own beliefs. Here there is a sense that such Jews fall victim to the drunkenness associated with civil society, with debauchery and with the lifestyle of the Christian fop.

Yet, within Friedländer's argument is the double sense that these rituals, such as drunkenness, if not the misreading of the Book of Esther itself, had once existed and had been eliminated, at least among the most enlightened of the Jews, those in Germany. The lack of sobriety of the Eastern Jews was still in need of strenuous reform, as Friedländer notes in 1816 when he was consulted by Malziewsky, Bishop of Kujawia, at the point when the Prussian government decided to improve the situation of the Polish Jews. (He published his report in 1819, with a title echoing that of Dohm's earlier tractate on German Jews: *On the Civic Improvement of the Jews of Poland*.) German Jews had become decorous, and abandoned crude practices that only masked the true religious significance of the Purim celebration. Jews in Germany were not drunkards, at least not in religious rituals that formed the public face of Jewish practice.

Friedländer was of course quite right that in his and the public's perception enlightened Jews were no longer drinking to excess. No less an authority on public decorum than the Königsberg philosopher Immanuel Kant (1724–1804) recognized this. In 1798, sitting down at the age of seventy-four to revise his lectures on 'anthropology'—originally delivered during the winter semester of 1772–3 but repeated as late as 1790–1—Kant added:

> Women, clergymen, and Jews normally do not get drunk, or at least they carefully avoid all appearance of it, because their civic status is weak and they need to be reserved (for which society is required). For their external worth rests simply on others' *belief* in their chastity, piety and separatistic lawfulness. For, as concerns the last point, all separatists, that is, those who submit themselves not only to a public law of the land but also to a special one (of their own sect), are, as oddities and alleged chosen people, particularly exposed to the attention of the community and the sting of criticism; thus cannot slacken their attention to themselves, since drunkenness, which removes caution, is a *scandal* for them.[60]

60 Immanuel Kant, *Anthropology from a Pragmatic Point of View*, trans. from the German by Robert B. Louden and Manfred Kuehn (Cambridge: Cambridge University Press 2006), 63–4 and Immanuel Kant, *Anthropologie in pragmatischer Hinsicht*, ed. Wilhelm Weischedel, in *Kant: Werke in Zehn Bände, Schriften zur Anthropologie, Geschichtsphilosophie, Politk und Pädagogik*, Zweiter Teil (Darmstadt: Wissenschaftliche Buchgesellschaft 1975), x.399–690 (all citations are to the pagination of the first edition ('A') as noted in this edition, which is identical with all other Kant editions: here A72–4). See E. M. Jellinek, 'Immanuel Kant on drinking', *Quarterly Journal of Studies of Alcohol*, vol. 1, 1941, 777–80. The view that Jews drink less because of their visibility as Jews is argued in 1947 by D. D. Glad, 'Attitudes and experiences of American-Jewish and American-Irish male youths as related to differences in adult rates of inebriety', *Quarterly Journal of Studies of Alcohol*, vol. 8, 1947, 406–72.

This is an addition to the first published version of the text in 1798. Kant summarizes the assumptions that underpin Friedländer's discussion of Bruns and his defence of the decorum of the German Jews. It is interesting that, in a further presentation of the Jews in his *Anthropologie*, Kant stresses, as does Knigge and all of the earlier Enlightenment thinkers, their nature as merchants and hagglers, and focuses particularly on the 'Jews in Poland'.[61] It is only in his discussion of Western Jews that he specifically returns to the question of decorum. Jews cannot afford to be visible in the public sphere as Jews, a point already made by Moses Mendelssohn in his insistence that Jews learn to speak the language of the nation in which they dwell. But the distinction here between public and private, with religious rite and practice being a private matter (as espoused by Mendelssohn), quickly shows itself to be specious. For Kant, they have ceased to act 'like savages' who, according to his views on madness in his lectures, have no control over their consumption of alcohol: 'The wildest peoples, as soon as they get to know strong drink, become desirous for it. People, who are indifferent to strong drink, very early succeed in rejecting this tendency.'[62] Jewish 'drunkenness' in terms of the eighteenth-century debate is an aspect of religious practice and does not directly impact on the public sphere in most cases. It is, however, seen as a reflection of inherent differences in religious practice that demand reform if Jews are to be seen as acceptable citizens in the public sphere. For all that the Jews do is pointless ritual. By Kant's day the inebriation of the German Jews had given way to the notion of Jewish sobriety in the use of alcohol. It is hypocritical for, like women and ministers of the cloth, it does not come from inner conviction but as a response to external forces. This change is one that is imagined as a process that took place in the late eighteenth century and—at least for Jewish thinkers such as Friedländer—was still not complete among Eastern Jews.[63]

The view, by the way, that Eastern Jews are prone to higher rates of alcoholism becomes a standard one in the course of the late nineteenth century when eugenicists in the United States, such as Emma Transeau, object to the presence of Eastern European Jews as a force in 'the

---

61 Kant, *Anthropologie*, A131n.
62 Immanuel Kant, *Immanuel Kant's Menschenkunde, oder philosophische Anthropologie. Nach handschriftlichten Vorlesungen*, ed. Friedrich Christian Starke (Leipzig: Die Expedition des europäischen Aufsehers 1831), 299.
63 The idea that Jewish 'sobriety' is a result of a historical process has been put forth in Mark Keller, 'The great Jewish drink mystery', *British Journal of Addiction*, vol. 64, 1970, 287–96, who dates its origins to the re-establishment of the Second Temple. Keller assumes a uniformity of modern Jewish experience and of this stereotype of the Jew as sober, but does understand this as part of a process of social change and adaptation. See also L. D. Hankoff, 'The roots of Jewish sobriety: alcoholism in the first century C.E.', *Koroth*, vol. 9, 1988, 62–72.

alcoholization of the immigrants' that will lead to American degeneration.[64] The common wisdom of the physicians by the turn of the century follows Kant. The British physician James Samuelson, in 1880, stated that 'they [the Jews] are a small community; and their partial isolation from other religious denominations has a tendency to make them more careful of their morals'.[65] Maurice Fishberg, the leading American exponent of Jewish public health at the turn of the century, argues, following Kant, that Jews have a much lower rate of alcoholism because they are subject to external social forces. This fitted nicely with his notion that,

> in their old home in Russia, the Jews abhor a drunkard; they name him with converts and outcasts. To have a drunkard in the family means difficulty in contracting suitable marriages for the children. The Jew knows that it does not pay to be drunk. Having lived for centuries under the ceaseless ban of abuse and persecution in the European Ghettoes, he has found it advantageous to his well being always to be sober.[66]

Yet Norman Kerr, at much the same time, advocated a genetic explanation:

> This extraordinary people has, amid wondrous vicissitudes, preserved a variety of distinctive characteristics; and I cannot help thinking that some inherited racial power of control as well as some inherited racial insusceptibility to narcotism, strengthened and confirmed by the practice of various hygienic habits, has been the main reason for their superior temperance.[67]

Or is it, following the model set by Knigge, only with 'the increased intercourse with non-Jews by the removal of social barriers' that there is 'an increase of alcoholism among Jews'?[68] As Fishberg noted in New York at the turn of the century, '... alcoholism is decidedly increasing among the Jews in New York, particularly in the younger generation, who are adapting the habits and customs of life of their gentile neighbors'.[69] By 1944 Robert Bales, in his Harvard dissertation and subsequent publication, holds the Eastern

64 Andrew Barr, *Drink: A Social History of America* (New York: Carroll and Graf 1999), 162.
65 James Samuelson, *A History of Drink: A Review, Social, Scientific, and Political* (London: Trübner and Co. 1878), 70–1.
66 Maurice Fishberg, *Health and Sanitation of the Immigrant Jewish Population of New York* (New York: Cowan 1902), 16. See his summary statement, Maurice Fishberg, *The Jews: A Study of Race and Environment*, 2 vols (New York: Harper 1949).
67 Norman Kerr, *Inebriety, Its Etiology, Pathology, Treatment and Jurisprudence* (London: H. K. Lewis 1889), 142, 145–6 (146).
68 Jacob Snowman, 'Jewish eugenics', *Jewish Review*, vol. 4, 1913–14, 159–74 (166). For French examples, see L. Chienisse, 'Rassenpathologie und Alkoholismus bei den Juden', *Zeitschrift für die Demographie und Statistik der Juden*, vol. 6, 1910, 1–8.
69 Fishberg, *Health and Sanitation of the Immigrant Jewish Population*, 18.

Jews up as the model immigrant community when it comes to alcohol use.[70] They have become the epitome of 'moderate, integrated, family based drinking', as opposed to Protestants who, if they drank, were much more likely to become alcoholics than Jews. If Kant's argument about Jewish moderation is based on the conscious anxiety of Jewish visibility, Bales accepts this, seeing alcoholism as the result of 'anxiety and repression', both of which he finds (in 1944!) much less prominent among Jews. One can add that, among Eastern European Jews, at least according to Maurice Samuels in 1943, it was the Russians who were 'stupid, perhaps, and earthy, given to drink and occasional wife-beating, but essentially good-natured'.[71] Everyone invents his or her own drunks.

Here we can return to the claims of the geneticists who argue that the presence of a specific genetic allele provides immunity against alcoholism for Jews. As the core 'evidence' for such claims is not physiological (flushing) but rather frequency of alcohol use based on self-reporting, we can select from a wide range of explanations from that of Kant to that of modern genetics to 'explain' the supposed absence of alcohol abuse. Indeed, one could imagine that there is little or no 'real' difference among the self-identified 'Jews' and any other cohort but that the stigma still lingering in American Jewish culture about alcohol abuse might modify the self-reporting. In fact, even physiological signs (such as flushing) could well have a psychological component. One needs to think about complex behaviours as a constant admixture of inherited and learned responses. This is at the core of the transition that the new genetics is being forced to make in regard to its inheritance of 'racial' categories, such as that of the 'Jews', from earlier stages of biological thought.

Sander L. Gilman is Distinguished Professor of the Liberal Arts and Sciences at Emory University in Atlanta. A cultural and literary historian, he is the author and editor of over seventy books. His biography *Franz Kafka* was published in 2005, and his most recent edited volume, a special issue of *History of Psychiatry* on 'Mind and Body in the History of Psychiatry' appeared in 2006.

---

70 Robert Bales, 'The "Fixation Factor" in Alcohol Addiction: A Hypothesis Derived from a Comparative Study of Irish and Jewish Social Norms', dissertation, Harvard University, 1944; Robert Bales, 'Cultural differences in rates of alcoholism', *Quarterly Journal of Studies of Alcohol*, vol. 6, 1946, 480–99.
71 Maurice Samuel, *The World of Sholom Aleichem* (New York: Alfred A. Knopf 1943), 131. Part of the literary image of the Eastern Jew in (at least) Polish literature is his role as a tavern keeper, keeping the peasants drunk in order to exploit them. See Magdalena M. Opalski, *The Jewish Tavern-Keeper and His Tavern in Nineteenth Century Polish Literature* (Jerusalem: Zalman Shazar Center for Jewish History 1986).

Reflections on race and the biologization of difference

KATYA GIBEL AZOULAY

ABSTRACT   In this article Gibel Azoulay critiques the tenacity of the correlation between 'race' as a socio-political notion and 'race' as a biological entity in academic circles in general and medical research in particular. Legacies of nineteenth-century scientific racism percolate into the public sphere, facilitating a uniquely US American cultural consensus that imagines and markets external physiological features as gross criteria for making distinctions, highlighting the medicalization of race in pharmaceutical, medical and genetic research.

Making sense of difference

Curiosity and concern about *difference* persist because, on the one hand, it informs the ways in which social entities (groups) imagine and recognize themselves as collectives and, on the other hand, it defines the boundaries across which groups (social entities) compete for recognition, rights and resources, the three-pronged grid of power. Community manifests itself as a collective and subjective experience that is projected through idioms of identity. In this context, the intuitive and visceral sense of belonging becomes a sentiment that is culturally comprehensible within the community and articulated through degrees of inclusion and exclusion. How we conceptualize *difference*—how we interact with, live alongside and integrate with it—is reflected in and thought through the corollary and opposite idea, *sameness*. These epistemological and philosophical concerns have been stretched to become epidemiological ones in biomedical research. My intention in this article, prefaced by reflections on the vocabulary of race and concluding with a critique of the metaphor *genetic signature*, is to consider the implications of thinking through the prism of 'difference' and 'race' in biomedical and genetic research while bearing in mind the following principle: the concept of 'race' cannot be sanitized, salvaged or made palatable.

In contrast to ancient Greek conceptions of difference, which were organized around geographic space, it is sight that has been privileged by

Europeans.[1] In order to explain human variation as the latter perceived it, a cohort of elite (white) European and (Anglo) American scientists invented a myth of 'race'. The racial typologies that they elaborated are, to borrow from Frantz Fanon, a white man's artefact that deserves to be archived rather than displayed.[2] The word 'race', as Ashley Montagu complained in his 1942 book *Man's Most Dangerous Myth*,[3] conveys and normalizes the idea of a resistant variety of natural difference. In the United States, the popular or commonsense understanding of 'race' correlates certain physical characteristics and lines of descent. 'Race' is imagined and lived on the fault lines of skin colour and ancestry, as well as in the collective memory of groups whose members share a history of exclusion, marginalization and oppression based only on the colour of their skin or ancestry.

The body, metaphorically read as a text, is subject to interpretations and translations because learning to *see* and to create meaning out of what is seen is context-bound and situational.[4] This is exemplified when brown- and black-skinned visitors to the United States, particularly from Latin America, feel misidentified if presumed to be 'black', graphically demonstrated by the results of the 2000 US Census in which a significant percentage of people who marked the Hispanic/Latino 'ethnic' category refused to identify themselves by race and did not identify themselves as 'white'.[5] A more instructive instance of learning to discern meaningful difference is demonstrated when foreigners who visited conflict-ridden Bosnia, Rwanda and Northern Ireland failed to *see* the differences combatants assumed were obvious, even though documents were often required to identify individuals. Perhaps the most incisive lesson about perception is in the following anecdote, shared by Patricia Williams, about an exchange in the 1930s between a Haitian statesman and an American official:

'What percent of Haiti's population is white?' asked the American. 'Ninety-five percent,' came the answer. The American official was flustered and, assuming

1 V. Y. Mudimbe, 'The power of the Greek paradigm', *South Atlantic Quarterly*, vol. 92, no. 2, 1993, 361–86.
2 Frantz Fanon, *Black Skin, White Masks* (New York: Grove Press 1967).
3 Ashley Montagu, *Man's Most Dangerous Myth: The Fallacy of Race* (New York: Columbia University Press 1942).
4 John Berger and Frantz Fanon offer very different but equally provocative explications of the social construction of seeing: John Berger, *Ways of Seeing* (London: Penguin 1972); Fanon, *Black Skin, White Masks*.
5 Mireya Navarro, 'Going beyond black and white, Hispanics in Census pick "Other"', *New York Times*, 9 November 2003, 1. Academic research and media analyses that explore the relationship of physical appearance (skin colour) and class to perceptions of racial identity within Latin America (including Brazil) report that, although colour prejudice and racism exist, it is conceptualized and articulated differently than in the United States. Consequently, immigrants to the US have to learn a new vocabulary, new ways of seeing and new ways of thinking that, in turn, impact on social interactions within immigrant communities as well as between immigrants and with Americans.

that the Haitian was mistaken, exclaimed, 'I don't understand—how on earth do you come up with such a figure?'

'Well, how do you measure blackness in the United States?'

'Anyone with a black ancestor.'

'Well, that's exactly how we measure whiteness,' retorted the Haitian.[6]

If race is a matter of perception, not biology, why does it continue to be used in biomedical research and genetic studies? And, if population groups are not products of nature but products of history—and therefore socially constituted and reconstituted on the basis of changing circumstances—who has the authority to delineate, define and name a group? For what purpose and on what basis?

Teaching at a residential liberal arts college has taught me the importance of directing student attention to the historical contexts within which authority validates knowledge as credible or acceptable. It has also made me appreciate being in the classroom, professing rather than protesting the significance of race as ideology, not biology, 'which came into existence at a discernible historical moment for rationally understandable historical reasons and is subject to change for similar reasons'.[7] No semester ends without a student complaining about a frustrating conversation about 'race' outside the classroom in which the attempt to share new understandings about the history of the concept is obstinately met with the insistence that '*race* is real, we can see it, we experience it, it's part of nature'. The argument that race is a social construction is dismissed as academic hyperbole, the evidence for this point provided by media reports of racial(ized) medical disorders and diseases.

In response, I point out that challenging ways of thinking is especially difficult when the terms 'race' and 'ethnicity' are routinely used in textbooks, academic texts, popular publications and the media as a shorthand reference for people.[8] Backed by such an arsenal of support, 'race' is not merely an abstract category of analysis but becomes part of the social vocabulary, signifying discrete populations distinguished by identifiable visible markers (phenotype). In the last forty years, the development of new technologies has enabled molecular biologists to study genotype (invisible markers). Research

6 Patricia Williams, *Seeing a Color-Blind Future: The Paradox of Race* (New York: Noonday Press 1998), 52.

7 Barbara Jeanne Fields, 'Slavery, race and ideology in the United States of America', *New Left Review*, no. 181, May–June 1990, 95–118 (101). See Fields's article on 'ideology' as a reference point for deeply rooted commonsense thinking; for a more comprehensive examination of the concept, see Terry Eagleton, *Ideology: An Introduction* (London: Verso 1991).

8 Barbara Jeanne Fields, 'Categories of analysis? Not in my book', in *Viewpoints: Excerpts from the ACLS Conference on Humanities in the 1990s*, American Council of Learned Societies Occasional Paper, no. 10 (New York: ACLS 1989), available online at www.acls.org/op10fields.htm (viewed 26 July 2006).

in this field should have exorcised the myth of biological race and pioneered radically new biocultural paradigms. Yet, despite molecular biology's promise of a more sophisticated examination of human variation beneath and beyond the surface of the skin, phenotype remains well within the repertoire of scientific speculation. As a category of analysis and a tool to differentiate populations, *difference* continues to be thought through the prism of race, which organizes population groups by appearance, geography and language and coincides with nineteenth-century racial typologies.[9]

The overlap of race, ethnicity and culture

When I send students to seek out encyclopaedia entries on 'race' and 'ethnicity', they return bewildered by the overlap between terms they assumed were distinct. As an example of this confusion, consider the following two definitions:

> The terms (ethnic groups, ethnicity) began to be used in the period immediately after World War II as a substitute for older terms as 'tribes' and (in British usage) 'race.'[10]

> The term 'ethnicity' is of recent origin and ... refers to both seeing oneself and being seen by others as part of a group on the basis of presumed ancestry and sharing a common destiny with others ... The common features may be racial (color), religious, linguistic, occupational or regional. The term 'ethnic group' appeared in part as a substitute for the words 'race' and 'tribe' and as a synonym for 'cultural group'.[11]

9 Appearance (phenotype), geography (continent and nationality) and invisible markers (genotype) all serve as surrogates for 'race' while, in turn, 'race' is used as a surrogate for biology. This underlines the question of whether purported correlates between genes and human population groups are based on prescriptive research in which researchers who identify these correlations are merely confirming, rather than casting doubt on, their expectations. In a special issue on race, the academic journal *Nature Genetics* included articles in which, as *New York Times* journalist Nicholas Wade reported, 'several geneticists wrote that people can generally be assigned to their continent of origin on the basis of their DNA, and that these broad geographical regions correspond to self-identified racial categories, such as African, East Asian, European and Native American. Race, in other words, does have a genetic basis, in their view.' That view was challenged by several Howard University scholars who countered that 'there was no biological basis for race and that any apparent link between genes and disease should be made directly, without taking race into account'. Nicholas Wade, 'Race-based medicine continued ...', *New York Times*, 14 November 2004.

10 Thomas Barfield (ed.), *The Dictionary of Anthropology* (Oxford and Cambridge, MA: Blackwell 1997).

11 Alan Barnard and Jonathan Spencer (eds), *Encyclopedia of Social and Cultural Anthropology* (London: Routledge 1996).

As the term 'ethnicity' gained widespread popularity, percolating from the academy into the public arena, its origins as a substitute for 'race' in response to Nazism faded from public memory. From the 1940s the term 'ethnic groups' in the United States became associated with groups previously thought of as European races that had blended politically into the melting pot of generic whiteness.[12] In contrast, 'race' became the term that signalled the ubiquitous line that divided Whites from 'Coloreds/ Negroes' (defined by having an African ancestor rather than by colour).[13] The first encyclopaedia entry above makes clear that 'ethnicity' was introduced to replace the terms 'race' and 'tribe'. This change occurred against the backdrop of anti-racist activities in the United States and anti-colonialist movements throughout Africa and Asia. Anthropologist Ashley Montagu, the staunchest advocate for banishing the word 'race' altogether, argued that 'ethnicity' was an ideal substitute because, as a new term, it was politically neutral. If scholars and lay people used 'ethnicity' (instead of 'race'), with its emphasis on environmental and social conditions as explanations for group differences, then the way they thought about difference would also change.[14]

12 Focusing on Asian Americans, Susan Koshy persuasively argues that racial vocabularies shift to ethnic ones as class mobility emerges, proving the elasticity of whiteness. Susan Koshy, 'Morphing race into ethnicity: Asian Americans and critical transformations of whiteness', *boundary 2*, vol. 28, no. 1, Spring 2001, 153–94.

13 For the alchemy of race, a process of whitening Irish, Eastern and Southern European immigrants initially perceived as inferior races polluting the white Anglo-Saxon racial integrity of the nation, see Matthew Frye Jacobson, *Whiteness of a Different Color: European Immigrants and the Alchemy of Race* (Cambridge, MA: Harvard University Press 1998). Note as well the absence of uniformity in legal definitions of who was a 'Negro' or 'colored person', as these were determined by state, not federal statutes.

14 Within the discipline of anthropology, racial categories were challenged in the early twentieth century as Euro-American nativism and European antisemitism gathered force, and scrutiny of Jewish difference, in particular, ceased to be perceived as a matter of benign scientific interest. For instance, Franz Boas spent considerable time evaluating the relationship between environment and biology in order to prove that *nurture*, not *nature*, was responsible for differences between new immigrants and white Euro-American citizens. His studies of Jewish immigrants from Eastern Europe and their children provided—unsurprisingly, with hindsight—clear evidence that a changed social environment, including new occupations, diets and new patterns of exercise, altered the bodies (physical type) of the newcomers from impoverished backgrounds as characterized by prevailing stereotypes in their countries of origin. There is no reason to obscure the obvious: Boas, however discretely and with whatever degree of self-consciousness, also had a personal stake in establishing legitimacy among colleagues who were quite open about their animosity towards Jews. See G. M. Morant, 'Racial theories and international relations', *Journal of the Royal Anthropological Institute of Great Britain and Ireland*, vol. 69, no. 2, 1939, 151–62, for a stringent critique of the imprecision of the race concept, its abusive contribution to racist propaganda and the irresponsible silence of anthropologists.

As the second encyclopaedia entry indicates, contrary to Montagu's hopes, 'ethnicity' did not replace or displace 'race'. In the United States, the semantic transition of European immigrants from white racial types to white ethnics erased all trace of the racial vocabulary and imagery, so central to nineteenth- and early twentieth-century discourses of difference,[15] from the national collective memory. At the same time, 'race' continued to be associated with the epidermal surface of the body: skin colour.[16] However, while 'ethnicity' added culture and heritage to its definition, it also remained anchored to ancestry and shared descent. Consequently, metaphors of roots, blood and common origin have bound it to the race concept it was meant to replace.

The problem is simple: in the matter of race, there is no such thing as 'getting it right'. There are no generic races precisely because race is a metaphor, a social construct: a human invention whose criteria for differentiation are neither universal nor fixed but have always been used to manage difference. 'Race', 'ethnicity' and 'culture' manifest themselves as metonyms that presuppose difference to be inherited. After all, one does not wake up in the morning and arbitrarily declare oneself to be Chinese, Cherokee or Chicano and seriously expect to be identified and recognized as such without some proof. And once recognition is contingent on evidence we are directed to the registry of socio-political and legal—not biological—affairs.[17] Let us turn to one scientific text whose authors try and fail to turn away from the race concept.

Writing on the relationship between 'ethnicity and drug therapy for hypertension', the authors begin by disclaiming conventional race categories because the usefulness 'of race or skin color' is limited: '... whites and blacks are neither genetically homogeneous, nor exclusive of each other's genetic traits'.[18] Having equated 'race' with skin colour, and tentatively cast doubt on the utility of race categories, they then retreat and inform us that 'recent advances in genetics have made it possible for researchers to compare the human genome across races', and point to the genetic pool in Africa that 'contains more variation than elsewhere', proving that 'most of the genetic difference between two individuals is because they are not the same person, rather than because they are of different races'.[19] 'Race', however, is not a shibboleth that the authors toss out; rather, they propose examining populations as 'ethnic groups'. Ethnicity, they argue, 'has incorrectly been used as a synonym for race. In fact, ethnicity is a multidimensional classification that encompasses shared origins, social

15 For one late nineteenth-century review of contemporary research on 'the races of Europe', see Carlos C. Closson, 'The races of Europe', *Journal of Political Economy*, vol. 8, no. 1, 1899, 58–88.

16 Jacobson, *Whiteness of a Different Color*.

17 Katya Gibel Azoulay, 'Outside our parents' house: race, culture and identity', *Research in African Literature*, vol. 27, no. 1, 1996, 129–42.

18 K. Amudha, L. P. Wong and A. M. Choy, 'Ethnicity and drug therapy for hypertension', *Current Pharmaceutical Design*, vol. 9, no. 21, 2003, 1691–701 (1691).

19 Ibid.

background, culture and environment'.[20] Setting aside their error about the term's history, they overlook 'shared origin' as the common denominator between the concepts of 'race' and 'ethnicity'. Predictably, the vocabulary becomes confused when articulating the focus of the research project: 'examining the *black–white* differences in physiological responses to pharmacological challenges that may provide a link between these models and known *ethnic differences* in drug responses'.[21]

Here we have an instance, and examples occur throughout the medical literature, in which a preference for 'ethnicity' over 'race' is a semantic change that fails to disrupt the kind of race-thinking that leads to a biological differentiation between Whites and Blacks. Like most scientific articles, there is no operational definition of 'Blacks' (also referred to as 'American Blacks' and 'African Americans') or 'Whites' (sometimes labelled 'Caucasians').[22] How are 'Blacks' and 'Whites' defined as subjects of medical research when aggregate race categories muddle science and ideology?[23] Although notions of racial

20 Ibid.
21 Ibid. (emphasis added).
22 Consider the 1928 conclusions of anthropologist Melville Herskovitz who estimated that, contrary to 'the general belief that the "pure" Negroes were the majority ... almost 80% show mixing with White or American Indian, or both stocks', while, in terms of ethnic diversity, a blending of African groups had occurred among the slave population in the United States. Melville J. Herskovitz, *The American Negro: A Study in Racial Crossing* (New York: Alfred A. Knopf 1928), 10; see also Gunnar Myrdal, *An American Dilemma: The Negro Problem and Modern Democracy* (New York: Harper 1944), 1205 and August Meier, 'The racial ancestry of the Mississippi College Negro' [1949], in *A White Scholar and the Black Community, 1945–1965: Essays and Reflections* (Amherst: University of Massachusetts Press 1992). Despite public rhetoric against miscegenation, sexual relations between Anglo-American men and black slave women were tolerated throughout the slave period since they added to the slave population, as evidenced by statutes regulating the status of children of slave women; see Sidney Kaplan, 'The miscegenation issue in the election of 1864', *Journal of Negro History*, vol. 34, no. 3, 1949, 274–343.
23 Consider the clarification of terminology in the ruling issued in *The People of the State of California* v. *George W. Hall* (1854). George Hall, 'a free white citizen' of California convicted of murder on the testimony of a Chinese witness, successfully appealed its admissibility before the Supreme Court of California. Judge Charles Murray delivered the opinion of the court: 'The word "Black" may include all Negroes, but the term "Negro" does not include all Black persons. ... In using the words, "No Black, or Mulatto person, or Indian shall be allowed to give evidence for or against a white person," the Legislature, if any intention can be ascribed to it, allowed the most comprehensive terms to embrace every known class or shade of color, as the apparent design was to protect the white person from the influence of all testimony other than of persons of the same caste. ... We are of the opinion that the words "White," "Negro," "Mulatto," "Indian," and "Black person," wherever they occur in our Constitution and laws, must be taken in their generic sense, and that ... the words "Black person" ... must be taken as contradistinguished from White and necessarily excludes all races other than the Caucasian.' The Chinese witness, Judge Murray concluded, was *generically* 'black'; therefore, his testimony was deemed inadmissible.

purity have been discredited, it is difficult to ignore their imprint when the social vocabulary of race is used so casually and carelessly in medical research.[24]

Let us return to the students in my class. It takes only a few weeks for students to learn about the history of classifying groups as well as the corollary evolution of a field of enquiry that defined 'race and racial typologies' as a respectable and requisite subject for study. It takes an entire semester or more for them to digest the full weight of the legacy of this history. Reading a random comparison of race categories used in the US Census between 1850s and 2005, and articles on 'race and racial typologies' from respected nineteenth-century journals such as the *Journal of the Anthropological Institute of Great Britain and Ireland*, provide concrete and compelling evidence of the changing criteria used 'to race' groups. Documents culled from a century of research on race challenge, and usually undermine, students' assumptions that races are a natural division of people and that these divisions are based on visible appearance. Not only do they discover the lack of consensus over the number of races that have been identified by scholars, but they are often shocked by the inconsistency of the criteria used to differentiate between populations. Confronted by the histories that conditioned the development of the science of race, students acquire a more skeptical perspective on theories that presuppose racial categories as a starting point for examining difference between groups of humans. The encyclopaedia assignment leads students to discover the trace of race in all the entries on ethnicity. Subsequently, they begin to pay closer attention to the way the terms surface in everyday conversation, academic discourse and the media. Very quickly they notice that unless 'race' and 'ethnicity' appear as self-evident and without definition, in scientific papers and presentations no less than in popular discourses.

Turning to an excerpt from an essay that advocates the use of race in pharmacological research, readers are confidently advised:

---

24 On three different visits to the pulmonary clinic at the University of Iowa Medical Center, the registration clerks entered 'White' or 'Other' into their database for my white-looking daughter despite the fact that I had written 'Black/African-American' on the registration form. Evidently the information I initially supplied was invariably edited after we left, for at each visit we repeated the same ritual of clarifying the race-category information. The irony is that the asthmatic symptoms for which my daughter was then being monitored were inherited from my Ashkenazi Jewish grandmother and/or my Afro-Cuban Jamaican father. The claim for scientific merit in a multiracial category in medical research ignores the reality that the genealogy of most human beings reflects diverse geographical and national points of origin, each of which have their own racializing inscriptions of difference. See Robert Young, *Colonial Desire: Hybridity in Theory, Culture and Race* (London: Routledge 1995).

there should be more—not less—study of how people of different *races* respond to drugs. While *ethnicity* can be an imperfect measure, understanding the interplay between *race* and drug efficacy could be a crucial tool in ferreting out the *genetic traits* that could one day allow researchers to better tailor drugs to individuals.[25]

In this passage, 'race' and 'ethnicity' are synonyms used to avoid repetition. Neither of these terms is a 'discursive category'; they are rather presented as a physiological entity. Hidden beneath the exterior surface of the body lurks a set of essential characteristics (genetic traits) awaiting discovery. Once 'ferreted out', they may be unique to that individual but—an example of the biologization of difference—the (re)search begins with a preconceived map of ethno-racial groups that are recognizable. Individuals are then assigned to groups based on socio-political preconceptions.[26] Even where self-identification is used and individuals assign themselves to groups, 'race' and 'ethnicity' are socio-political, not biological, categories.

Molecular biology and genetic studies should have undermined the scientific validity of using any exterior cues to read the body and, perhaps more significantly, should have sent scientists back to the drawing board for more insightful ways to delineate population groups for study. Although genetic studies are promoted as a new field attentive to genetic codes that invalidate race as biology, the concept of 'race' continues to be deployed as an organizer of difference. Stuart Hall compellingly attributes this durability to the need for a guarantee of truth.[27] The problem is prescriptive, rather than open-ended, research: researchers begin by looking for genetic markers of population groups

25 Amy Barrett, 'Color-blind drug research is myopic', *Business Week*, 27 June 2005, 44 (emphasis added).
26 A relatively banal instance appears in a project on sensitivity to pain in which the researchers note the prevailing hypothesis that genetic factors contribute to pain. They organize their research according to pre-existing social categories of ethnicity in order to compare the effects of stimuli on different groups. The project involved 'a total of 500 normal participants (306 females and 194 males)', comprised of '62.0% European American, 17.4% African American, 9.0% Asian American, and 8.6% Hispanic, and 3.0% individuals with mixed racial parentage'. Not only are each of these social categories treated as discrete genetic entities, but even 'Hispanic' is treated as a generic race category. Predictably, the conclusions conform to and confirm the racial typology: 'Our observations demonstrate that gender, ethnicity and temperament contribute to individual variation in thermal and cold pain sensitivity. K. Hyungsuk, John K. Neubert, Anitza San Miguel, Ke Xu, Raj K. Krishnaraju, Michael J. Iadarola, David Goldman and Raymond Dionne, 'Genetic influence on variability in human acute experimental pain sensitivity associated with gender, ethnicity and psychological temperament', *Pain*, vol. 109, no. 3, June 2004, 488–96.
27 *Race: The Floating Signifier*, video recording, featuring Stuart Hall, produced, directed and edited by Sut Jhally (Northampton, MA: Media Education Foundation 1996).

and then correlate them to familiar ethnic and racial phenotypes.[28] Removing the certainty of biological race necessitates alternative explanations of difference. To move in this direction is to move away from any guarantee of truth.

Distinguishing social fact from biological fiction

The startling announcement that the Food and Drug Administration had approved a new heart drug specifically targeting black Americans was a reminder that race continues to be viewed as a viable biological variable among the science community, despite its history as an invention by eighteenth-century naturalists who were classifying everything they could see in order to make sense of their world. In that era of slavery and European colonial expansion, the presumption that humans could be divided according to visible physical characteristics seemed to correlate with divisions according to geographical areas and technological differences. Aesthetic and political biases informed the classification of human populations as species, later revised as a hierarchy of racial types ranked by degrees of civilization. By the mid-1800s the science of race had gained momentum as a prestigious field within which to study racial typologies. Cranial capacity as a measurement of intelligence, as well as shape of nose, feet, ears and other parts of the body, were used to identify racial status, deviance, moral incorrigibility and servility. Metaphors of 'hybridity' connected biology with botany to signify a physiological phenomenon with political and cultural implications while heterosexual unions in the colonies, between colonizers and colonized, challenged theories of repugnance, infertility and degenera-

28 Unsuccessful efforts to find substantive differences between racial groups, where 'race' is defined by skin colour, have not led researchers to conclude that this kind of enquiry should be abandoned. In an article reviewing findings on racial differences in skin pathophysiology, the authors conclude that more—not less—research is needed because 'we still cannot answer the question, "how resistant is black skin compared with white?"'; Enzo Berardesca and Howard Maibach, 'Racial differences in skin pathophysiology', *Journal of the American Academy of Dermatology*, vol. 34, no. 2, 1996, 667–72. Hu *et al.* claim evidence for their conclusion that 'difference in the incidence of uveal melanoma between each racial/ethnic group was highly statistically significant, with the exception of the black versus the Asian population in which there was no statistically significant difference'; D. N. Hu, G. P. Yu, S. A. McCormick, S. Schneider and P. T. Finger, 'Population-based incidence of uveal melanoma in various races and ethnic groups', *American Journal of Ophthalmology*, vol. 140, no. 4, October 2005, 612–17. See also Melbourne Tapper's study of the tenacity with which scientists correlated sickle cell anaemia with ethnological categories, characterizing the medical disorder as a 'black disease'. Confronted by evidence to the contrary, explanations were offered linking patients to migrations from Africa that occurred several centuries earlier; Melbourne Tapper, *In the Blood: Sickle Cell Anemia and the Politics of Race* (Philadelphia: University of Pennsylvania Press 1999).

tion. Racial discourse highlighted the centrality of power in its politicization of sex, illustrated in British concerns over mixed-race people in India and South Africa, and fuelled debates in the United States over the annexation of Mexico. Finally, litigation in US courts over the racial status of individuals testified to the contradictions of racial categories as the criteria were consistently unstable and unreliable.[29]

This brief overview highlights 'race' as an academic fiction that took root as an ideology of difference and served to rationalize, buttress and justify discriminatory legislative and political policies. Although today most scientists no longer attempt to correlate racial difference with innate mental characteristics or value systems, the belief that race refers to measurable physiological differences is still promoted as credible. One recent and astounding example is a pilot study that examined

> multivariate craniofacial anthropometric distributions between biologically ad-mixed male populations and single racial groups of Black and White males. Multivariate statistical results suggested that nose breadth and lip length were different between Blacks and Whites. Such differences may be considered for adjustments to respirators and chemical-biological protective masks. However, based on this pilot study, multivariate anthropometric distributions of admixed individuals were within the distributions of single racial groups. Based on the sample reported, *sizing and designing for the admixed groups are not necessary if anthropometric distributions of single racial groups comprising admixed groups are known*.[30]

Reports in both the media and academic journals on race and medicine fail to specify the criteria used to determine racial classification although it is reasonable to suggest that researchers and readers assume that groups studied or tested in clinical trials are classified by popular notions of race with concordance between appearance and self-identification. Consequently, reports about the positive impact of BiDil on 'Blacks' and 'African Americans' relied on the presumption of visibly brown-skinned individuals rather than explicit information on the criteria used to determine who was Black or African American. This is a serious oversight. Given the diverse

29 On the variety of courtroom arguments and legal strategies used to control racial ambiguity and maintain racial difference, see Ariela J. Gross, 'Litigating whiteness: trials of racial determination in the nineteenth-century South', *Yale Law Journal*, vol. 108, no. 1, October 1998, 109–80; Michael Elliott, 'Telling the difference: nineteenth-century legal narratives of racial taxonomy', *Law & Social Inquiry*, vol. 24, no. 3, 1999, 611–36; and John Tehranian, 'Performing whiteness: naturalization litigation and the construction of racial identity in America', *Yale Law Journal*, vol. 109, no. 4, January 2000, 817–46.

30 M. Yokota, 'Head and facial anthropometry of mixed-race US Army male soldiers for military design and sizing: a pilot study', *Applied Ergonomics*, vol. 36, no. 3, May 2005, 379–83 (emphasis added).

ancestral backgrounds of most Americans of African descent—including both European and American Indian ancestors—as well as the 'forgotten' ancestry of some self-identified white Americans—those whose ancestors 'passed' for white, Spanish or Indian—it seems distinctly *unscientific* to rely on either self-identification or observation as the primary criterion for determining physiological differences. NitroMed's decision to test BiDil on self-identified Blacks, and its subsequent conclusion that the drug proved more effective in them than in Whites reinforced the validity of considering 'race' as a biological concept. This created both a pedagogical opportunity and a challenge for educators who teach that race and racial categories are simultaneously a social fact and a biological fiction.

Commonplace ideas about race register the gross physical features of the body that serve as templates for the stories and metaphors that compose meaningful difference. The ideologies that give substance to ideas of racial distinction ignore or overlook more durable and immutable variables, such as digestive enzymes and blood types, as criteria for constructing typologies used to study groups of people.[31] Switching from 'race' to such typologies requires a perceptual and conceptual transformation of scientists and social scientists working in different areas of population studies. Instead, the presumption of an essential immutable 'racial' distinction, reflected in claims about the unique effectiveness of BiDil on 'African Americans', conveniently deflects attention away from societal factors that cause cardiovascular disease. Rather than attribute the *appearance* of 'race-based' differential responses to 'race', a more responsible approach would be to examine differences in the physiological impact of living in a *racialized* society in which apparent difference between population groups are a consequence of different experiences with racism, racial discrimination and both overt and covert prejudice. The biologization of race is not just bad politics but also bad science. Though criticized by some scientists, the tautological use of 'race', in which it is informed by and reproduces *racialized truths*, remains deeply embedded in 'ritualized scientific practice'.[32]

Debates over advertising BiDil as 'an ethnic drug' again revealed the overlap between the terms 'ethnicity' and 'race'. More importantly, they centred around the question of whether race has epidemiologic utility. Opponents urged more attention to racism as a substantial negative health factor impacting Blacks differently than Whites. While Sharon Wyatt *et al.* argued that comparative research on rates of cardiovascular disease among different social groups should begin with the differential effect of institutionalized racism, Jules Harrell *et al.* presented supporting evidence that direct

31 Stephen Jay Gould, 'The geometer of race', *Discover*, vol. 15, no. 11, November 1994, 64–9.
32 Sandra Soo-Jin Lee, Joanna Mountain and Barbara A. Koenig, 'The meanings of "race" in the new genomics: implications for health disparities research', *Yale Journal of Health Policy, Law and Ethics*, vol. 1, Spring 2001, 33–75.

encounters with discriminatory events contributed to negative health out-comes.[33] An alternative to the presupposition of a correlation between race and biology might be the question of whether the stress of racism leads to medical disorders in ways that are analogous to the stress of noise-level or sitting in traffic. If these stresses are analogous, a more efficient approach might be to identify and examine racism as a risk factor that explains race-based disparities in cardiovascular disease. If this is the starting point, then race as a *social* fact does indeed have epidemiologic utility. In fact, this is hardly a novel idea: the link between racism and health was pioneered by psychiatrist and political theorist Frantz Fanon in the field of psychiatry when he identified colonialism as the causal agent for most of the psychological disorders of his patients, and prescribed its overthrow as the cure. Until racism is placed under the microscopic gaze of medical and genetic research, we will not know whether health-related disorders currently over-represented in the population identified as Black/African American are a result of racism or the experience of *being raced*.

Popularizing the myth of race

Though it may be a truism to note the significant role television plays as a conduit of information and misinformation, it is nevertheless worthy of attention as the following example shows. Several months ago, I watched an episode of the popular crime scene investigation series *CSI*. The central theme of this episode focused on the murder of a thirteen-year-old girl who had been intentionally conceived by her parents as a medical resource for their only son who suffered from a deadly and rare disease that required a matching blood type. Over the years, the daughter donated her blood and bone marrow but the sorry situation escalated until her brother needed a kidney transplant. The daughter was designated to be the donor in yet another painful medical procedure. But, as a normal teenager who wanted to have fun rather than be confined to a hospital bed, she began to express reservations, much to the chagrin of her mother. The investigation concluded with the revelation that the brother killed his sister to save her from another medical ordeal on his behalf. So much for the plot.

  CSI is among a number of television programmes that intentionally convey information on health-related issues. This episode identified the

33 Sharon B. Wyatt, David R. Williams, Rosie Calvin, Frances C. Henderson, Evelyn R. Walker and Karen Winters, 'Racism and cardiovascular disease in African Americans', *American Journal of the Medical Sciences*, vol. 325, no. 6, June 2003, 315–31; Jules P. Harrell, Sadiki Hall and James Taliaferro, 'Physiological responses to racism and discrimination: an assessment of the evidence', *American Journal of Public Health*, vol. 93, no. 2, February 2003, 243–8.

main characters as a 'mixed-race' couple, a Latino father and his white American wife, which set the context for describing their children as 'racially mixed'. Relying on commonsense notions about distinctions between social groups, this representation of marriage across socially defined racial lines reinforced the premise that 'race' is more than a social category and experience: 'race' from this perspective is located within the body. Consequently, the logic behind the episode, which made the plot culturally comprehensible to its American audience, necessarily relied on a biological understanding of 'race' as well as a mistaken assumption that the label 'Hispanic/Latino' refers to a racial group.[34]

The script left no doubt that the CSI team judged the actions of the parents as morally repugnant. Yet, despite the message that it is wrong to conceive a child as a medical repository for a sibling, a more discrete and compelling message was communicated to viewers in a forceful statement articulated by the (white) mother. They were not cruel parents, she argued, and defended their actions by pointing to the absence of 'mixed-race' donors who might have helped to save the life of their son. Viewed from this perspective, they faced a serious dilemma. However abhorrent, the script offered viewers a narrative in which the medical challenges facing a 'mixed-race' couple are different than those of 'same-race' couples.

This particular CSI episode dramatizes the success that proponents of an official 'multiracial' census category have had. The most assertive of these organizations, Project Race, was established in 1991 by Susan Graham, a white woman married to a black man, who did not want to list her children as either 'white' or 'black'. Through aggressive campaigning, recruitment and outreach programmes, Project Race was propelled under Graham's leadership into the centre of debates over racial categories listed on the US Census. Although a multiracial category was not included in the 2000 Census, many institutions and other agencies that collect demographic information now do include either a 'mixed-race' category, an opportunity to mark more than one racial category or an 'other' category, indicating that

34 The CSI script reinforces the misuse of 'Hispanic' as a racial term. In fact, as the only official 'ethnic' category on the US Census, 'Latino/Hispanic' registers the population of Mexico, Central and South America The official, though informal, recognition of the diverse mix of African, indigenous and European ancestries in Spanish-speaking countries disappears when 'Latino/Hispanic' is treated as a generic race category. Moreover, as David Hayes-Bautista points out in relation to academic research, definitional differences and confusion of terminology have led to inconsistent or conflicting research methodologies and conclusions. As a political issue, this confusion has significant consequences for policy, especially in terms of access to benefits guaranteed under remedial civil rights legislation. David E. Hayes-Bautista, 'Identifying "Hispanic" populations: the influence of research methodology upon public policy', American Journal of Public Health, vol. 70, no. 4, April 1980, 353–6.

more than one racial category applies to the registering individual.[35] Project Race, according to its mission statement, 'advocates for multiracial children and adults through education, community awareness and legislation. Our main goal is for a multiracial classification on all school, employment, state, federal, local, census and medical forms requiring racial data.'[36]

The Project Race website identifies 'urgent medical concerns' as the most compelling factor in its crusade for justice, listing a series of 'facts' that purportedly identify special issues facing 'multiracial children', including their omission from health statistics and pharmaceutical clinical trials. Its most noteworthy claim, that 'there is a shortage of bone marrow donors for the multiracial population',[37] is reiterated in the *CSI* episode that, in turn, disseminates to a broad audience the fallacious claim that 'multiracial' people are an identifiable and distinct group that can, and should, be distinguished from other 'racial groups'.[38] Project Race was followed by the establishment of other organizations for 'mixed-raced persons', one of which, the MAVIN Foundation, also supports the claim that 'multiracial people have great difficulty finding marrow or blood stem cell matches to cure potentially fatal diseases like leukemia'.[39] It initiated the MatchMaker Bone Marrow Project, which 'is the only national program dedicated to mixed race bone marrow donor recruitment and education'.[40] The problem is that the notion of 'mixed-race persons' is necessarily based on prior racialization. These identity-based organizations do not instruct the public about a changing *sociological* dynamic but rather reinforce the premise that race is biological: the presumption of discrete racial groups enables *amalgamation* and *admixture*. This differentiation of population groups on the basis of biological criteria conveniently, and sometimes deliberately, ignores the unstable history of the race concept and the evolution of race as an ideology.

35 Cautioning that conclusions based on current methods of collecting race/ethnicity data are inconsistent because of a 'lack of consensus and inadequate definitions for terminology; and misclassification or miscounting of patients', two researchers argue for a more detailed set of categories, including 'mixed-heritage', an example of the persistent effort to improve rather than invalidate racial taxonomies. P. Davis and L. Rubin, 'Obstruction of valid race/ethnicity data acquisition by current data collection instruments', *Methods of Information in Medicine*, vol. 37, no. 2, June 1998, 188–91.

36 'Mission statement', available on the Project Race website at www.projectrace.com/aboutprojectrace/ (viewed 11 September 2006).

37 'The health status of multiracial Americans fact sheet', available on the Project Race website at www.projectrace.com/urgentmedicalconcern/ (viewed 11 September 2006).

38 Davis and Rubin, 'Obstruction of valid race/ethnicity data acquisition by current data collection instruments'.

39 Homepage of MatchMaker, a MAVIN project, at www.mavin.net/Matchmaker.html (viewed 29 July 2006).

40 Ibid. MatchMaker was founded in 2001 by two interns to address the 'chronic shortage of multiracial donors on the NMDP [National Marrow Donor Program]'.

The pervasive reiteration of 'race' as a noun—an entity that can be isolated and measured as an object of study—obfuscates the role of racism in shaping experiences that give race its salient visceral and cognitive potency. Advocates of a multiracial category, as well as media references to multiracial people, consistently disregard, and persistently omit, the oft-repeated qualifications, which are carefully interspersed throughout the Office of Management and Budget (OMB) policy directive that clarifies the race categories included on the federal Census document (as well as how the data are to be tabulated and used). Given the considerable amount of misinformation that circulates in the public domain as well as continuing demands to increase the number of categories on the next Census, it is appropriate to quote directly from this document:

> Development of the data standards [on race and ethnicity] stemmed in large measure from new responsibilities to enforce civil rights laws. Data were needed to monitor equal access in housing, education, employment, and other areas, for populations that historically had experienced discrimination and differential treatment because of their race or ethnicity. The standards are used not only in decennial census (which provides the data for the 'denominator' for many measures), but also in household surveys, on administrative forms (e.g., school registration and mortgage lending applications), and in medical and other research. *The categories represent a social-political construct designed for collecting data on the race and ethnicity of broad population groups in this country, and are not anthropologically or scientifically based.*[41]

It is certainly true that this passage precedes a statement that the categories 'should not be interpreted as being *primarily biological or genetic* in reference' (emphasis added), which seems to contradict the earlier acknowledgment that they are 'a social-political construct'. Furthermore, the following comment that 'race and ethnicity may be thought of in terms of social and cultural characteristics as well as ancestry' also suggests that race categories overlap genealogy (ancestry) and genes (biology). Does the contradiction indicate uncertainty within OMB over the relationship between 'race' as a social construct and 'race' as a biological phenomenon? Or is this a misleading over-interpretation that deflects attention from the insistence that the categories intentionally register the legacy of distinctions within populations residing in the United States that have been subject to adverse differentiation and discrimination?

---

41 US Census Bureau, Office of Management and Budget, 'Revisions to the standards for the classifications of federal data on race and ethnicity', 30 October 1997 (last modified 2 November 2000), available at www.census.gov/population/www/socdemo/race/Ombdir15.html (viewed 29 July 2006) (emphasis added).

Race and grammar

'Race' is sensible only as a predicate, an action verb that requires an agent and intention. A person, persons or policies drafted by persons 'race' individuals and groups. 'Racing' produces the social fact that informs experience. Consequently, when 'racing' is embedded in the fabric of everyday life, it is normalized and functions as an ideology (common sense). 'Racing' under these circumstances is durable as part of the *habitus*, a predisposition that does not require conscious thought.[42] In its more popular form, however, 'race' is deployed as a noun and presumes fundamental physiological differences between groups of people. Arguments over whether race is 'real' hinge on whether it is understood as an action verb or a self-evident noun. When 'race' is used as a verb, racism insinuates itself into discussions whereas, when expressed as a noun, racism escapes attention and therefore can be ignored.

Let me be clear: thinking difference, usefully conceptualized by means of the philosophical paradigm of Self and Other, is not inherently antagonistic and, therefore, the observation of markers that differentiate one person from another is, in principle, benign. In contrast, thinking in terms of 'race-based' differences is learned and informed by a discriminating distinction whose origins can be traced to a specific era and set of events. This can best be appreciated by recalling a pivotal moment in the history of bondage in the United States. In 1662 the colony of Virginia passed its first statute on the question of status and 'the Negro', and the language is particularly relevant:

> Whereas some doubts have arisen whether children got by an Englishman upon a negro woman should be slave or free. Be it therefore enacted and declared by this present grand assembly, that all children borne in this country shall be held bond or free only according to the condition of the mother.[43]

It is clear that the statute was passed because there was a problem with English men having sexual relations with women of African descent. Since these were the only women indentured for life, there was no reason to include Englishwomen in the statute although ambiguity was removed by qualifying 'woman' with the adjective 'negro'. The catalyst behind this statute was neither concern about sex across the colour line nor about sex between free persons and the enslaved. Instead, the legislators were motivated by concerns about property, not propriety.

42 Pierre Bourdieu, *Language and Symbolic Power*, ed. John B. Thompson, trans. from the French by Gino Raymond and Matthew Adamson (Cambridge, MA: Harvard University Press 1991).
43 A. Leon Higgenbotham, Jr., *In the Matter of Color: Race and the American Legal Process: The Colonial Period* (Oxford: Oxford University Press 1980), 44.

Legislative intervention into the private sphere of heterosexual relations explicitly addressed the consequences of impregnating slave women who gave birth. In a society in which enslaved human beings were possessions, codification of property rights was both reasonable and logical. From a seventeenth-century perspective, distinguishing between free and slave in the English colonies was an economic problem that had to be definitively resolved. Reframed as a legal problem, it was necessary to reverse English laws of inheritance that were determined by paternal descent, and legislate maternal descent as the criterion determining the status of bondage and freedom. This revision was expressly designed to protect slave-owners' property. It is therefore noteworthy that the legislators who crafted the statute did not raise or address the question of whether the child would be a 'negro' or 'English'. Such finer distinctions required the intervention of scientific racism. As long as slavery was part of a worldview that took inequality and hierarchy for granted, there was no reason for a racial ideology.[44] Only when freedom became a doctrine and human perfectibility became a philosophical postulate was an explanation for slavery required. In the United States the association of permanent servitude—slavery—and 'Negroes' cemented the presumption of a relation between colour and physiology.[45]

The history of racial theory is crucial and needs to be incorporated in undergraduate introductory courses in general, and the sciences in particular, if students are to grasp the profound connection between 'race', 'ethnicity' and 'culture' as concepts that are neither neutral nor innocent. Racial theories began in the academy in a discourse literally invented by anthropologists, linguists, philosophers and members of the medical profession at the same time that professionalization of the sciences was taking place. The data they assembled and disseminated provided an essential supplement to prejudice and were thus an important basis for formulating, rationalizing and enacting government policies and legislative decisions. Furthermore, racial classifications evolved within two areas of study: physiology and language.

44 On predominantly servant immigration from Europe, comprised of convicts and indentured servants, and their visibility within the colonies, see Aaron S. Fogleman, 'From slaves, convicts, and servants to free passengers: the transformation of immigration in the era of the American Revolution', *Journal of American History*, vol. 85, no. 1, June 1998, 43–76.

45 Certainty of the relation between colour and status was disrupted in the years before the Civil War when an increasing presence of white-skinned slaves who looked like their owners (and thus revealed paternity) testified to discrepancies in which visible markers might not be readily apparent. Note as well W. E. B. Du Bois's disparaging remark: 'The rape which your gentlemen have done against helpless black women in defiance of your own laws is written on the foreheads of two millions of mulattoes and written in ineffaceable blood' (quoted in Myrdal, *An American Dilemma*, 1187n14). See also Kaplan, 'The miscegenation issue in the election of 1864'.

Barbara Fields describes the intervention of science, biology and physical anthropology as 'the heavy artillery' that settled the conflict between the ideologies of equality (philosophical and religious) and racism.[46] Interest in understanding the origins and causes of superiority and inferiority prescribed scientific enquiry and predetermined conclusions of research that identified racial types and then examined the relationship between their physiological and mental characteristics. Robert Young defines the ideology of race as 'a semiotic system in the guise of ethnology, the science of races'. In his excellent book *Colonial Desire: Hybridity in Theory, Culture and Race*, Young highlights the 1820s, when linkages between European languages and Sanskrit elevated Asians to proximity with Caucasians and simultaneously opposed European languages to Semitic ones. This 'transformed the mere taxonomy of ethnograpy' by means of a

> genetic emphasis on the metaphor of 'families' of languages and the oft charted language 'trees' ... [These] were to determine the whole basis of phylogenetic racial theories of conquest, absorption and decline—designed to deny the more obvious possibilities of mixture, fusion and creolization.[47]

In other words: we have inherited a set of racial theories that articulated an anxious need to rationalize separation even as interaction and mixing were producing new people that defied and refuted the theories under construction. From this point, as Young astutely demonstrates, we are confronted by a complicated and contradictory history in which physical racial characteristics are allied to language families that in turn condition the emergence of a cultural system for classification and differentiation.[48]

Unlearning race

How do we undo race-thinking? The power of expertise and authority manifests itself in peer-reviewed academic journals that have a prominent stature in their discipline. This power reaches beyond academic circles and percolates into the public arena through the media whose reports discretely validate research conclusions as scientific even when these are subject to

46 'Presentation given by historian Barbara J. Fields at a "school" for the producers of RACE', March 2001, available under 'History' in 'Background Readings' on the website for the PBS series *Race—The Power of An Illusion* at www.pbs.org/race/ 000_General/000_00-Home.htm (viewed 11 September 2006).

47 Young, *Colonial Desire*, 65.

48 The ubiquitous connection between culture and colour is pronounced when the social vocabulary of race and socially defined racial markers of identity coincide and a social formation is identified and defined as 'cultural'. There is no better example, at least in the United States, to the way reference to 'culture' reinscribes boundaries than the essentialist ideas of what constitutes 'blackness' and 'whiteness'.

debate, as in the case of BiDil. Genetic researchers articulate their hypotheses in scientific language that has the semblance of unemotional authority. But as historians of science have elaborated, science as a practice and a discipline is neither objective nor neutral. Scientists are not expected to foreground conscientiously the cultural contexts within which their scientific curiosity, observations and hypotheses take shape when they present their findings and interpretations.[49]

The presumption of education, credentials and publication seems to preclude media analysis of the production of knowledge, the process of making information. Yet the relationship between researchers as practitioners, the pharmaceutical companies as profit-making institutions and the Food and Drug Administration's role in prescriptive policymaking is noteworthy. This three-way relationship has come under public scrutiny when abstract epistemological questions coincide with practical and politically sensitive policies. Critics who denounced the credibility of marketing a race-based drug pointed to the profit that NitroMed stood to gain by targeting African Americans as consumers, particularly given measurable racial inequality within the health care system that has underserved this population. While identifying Blacks as a social group whose experiences with varying degrees of racial discrimination—perceived and tangible—has merit for studying the physiological reactions to the cumulative effect of living in the United States, conflating genetics and social race facilely ignores racism while overplaying the finding that 'Blacks may produce less nitric oxide'.[50]

Four centuries of racism in the United States, propelled by an explicit strategy of maintaining white privilege and protecting white interests, has resulted in the naturalization of the principle of racial classifications constructed and modified within the unfolding field of anthropology. Although the specific criteria invoked to differentiate between classifications have changed over time, this principle of distinctions has retained its power. There can be little disagreement that health is always a major concern and that, therefore, research on health-related issues is, quite obviously, both indispensable and valuable. It is also understandable that the investigation of various medical problems would consider patterns within and between population groups in order to identify causes that would, in turn, enable remedial treatment. In other words, health-related research is motivated by very specific objectives and *desiderata*. What is not always obvious, however,

49 Paul Root Wolpe, 'If I am only my genes, what am I? Genetic essentialism and a Jewish response', *Kennedy Institute of Ethics Journal*, vol. 7, no. 3, September 1997, 213–30.

50 Kendra Lee, 'New drug may get to the heart of the problem', *The Crisis*, vol. 112, no. 1, January/February 2005, 12; David Rotman, 'Race and medicine', *Technology Review*, vol. 108, no. 4, April 2005, 60–5; D. R. Rutledge, Lavoisier Cardozo and Joel Steinberg, 'Racial differences in drug response: isoproterenol effects on heart rate in healthy males', *Pharmaceutical Research*, vol. 6, no. 2, February 1989, 182–5.

is the extent to which researchers import their social and political perspectives into their research. If white researchers are now over-compensating for ignoring Blacks in clinical studies, some black researchers are over-zealous in highlighting Blacks as subjects for research. In both cases, the use of 'race' as an organizing principle is evidence that conceptualizing populations along bogus racial lines persists as a respectable practice.

Using 'racial' as a keyword, an online search for articles in the Medline database for 2004–5 produced over 1,800 titles. Browsing through most of them, an admittedly time-consuming task, I was overwhelmed by comparisons that presumed that populations could be divided by racial groups as well as the apparent consensus among scholars over the composition of these groups. A random selection of articles were written in specialized scientific language appropriate to the field but obscure to the lay reader; it did not take a translator, however, to understand the a priori identification of race as an observable characteristic and to deduce, where it was not specific, that the primary mark of distinction between Whites and Blacks was skin colour.[51] In sum, even where there was a brief discussion of how 'race' was employed in the research, it was explicitly equated with appearance, without reference to the more likely hybrid composition of each population group examined in the respective study, particularly 'African Americans', 'Latinos' and 'Native Americans'. Regardless of how a respondent identifies him/herself, it is troubling that researchers assume, rather than question, the utility of using 'race' as a variable for physiological comparisons between populations.

As long as the fiction of race that has so influenced the discipline of anthropology permeates scientific research, race-thinking will be reproduced, naturalized in conversation and reinscribed through repetition in laboratory reports, conference papers, professional journals and in the classroom. Precisely because race is referenced as something physiological and then used as to compare groups raced as distinct with regard to such medical phenomena as iron deficiency, colorectal cancer, dementia and pulse pressure, it warrants attention and refutation whether or not one possesses the credentials that guarantee an audience.

What is needed is a reconceptualization of populations, and comparative studies that focus attention on more significant physiological differences determined by body chemistry, such as lactose tolerance or blood groups. Even if one grants latitude to analyses that use racial categories, the mandate

51 Like the current socially relevant categories on the US Census, 'African American' is used interchangeably with 'Black', 'Caucasian' is synonymous with 'White', and the geographical label of 'Asian' relies on the assumption of regional distinction as well as appearance. While some authors note in passing that racial categories are problematic, they nevertheless identify race as a credible factor to be examined in relation to other physiological and environmental variables. The most undefined and ambiguous category is 'Latino', a late twentieth-century renaming of 'Hispanic'; see Hayes-Bautista, 'Identifying "Hispanic" populations'.

should be that researchers explain both the use of such categories in the research as social—not biological—constructs as well as the fact that the categories used by researchers and patients inherently reflect an experienced social distinction. In contrast, differentiating populations on a mythical basis of race—even, and especially, when 'ethnicity' is imported as a more polite substitute for 'race', which only returns through the back door—registers belief in an 'essence' that is apparent in skin, hair texture and facial features.[52]

As a last example of the *medicalization* of race and the dissemination of misleading information to the public, consider advertisements and over-the-counter medications for osteoporosis in which labels identify 'Caucasian and Asian women' as particularly susceptible to bone fragility. The term 'Caucasian', coined by naturalist Johannes Blumenbach at the end of the eighteenth century (*Varietas Caucasia*), referred to the people living in the Caucasus region. When I introduce a new class of students to this history each semester, they are collectively taken aback to learn that 'Caucasian' became, in American English, a generic synonym for 'white' relatively recently. This detail has received considerable attention in articles and books about race and, though it is easily found in a quick Internet search, it nevertheless always strikes students as new information primarily because it does not circulate widely in the public sphere. This synonymity was predicated on the science of race that helped popularize 'Caucasian' as a generic term for white-skinned Europeans. 'Caucasian', as a racial type and category, was a necessary condition for prompting a shift in *conceptualizing* degrees of whiteness to a *perception* of physiological similarity. But, if thinking about skin colour as evidence of an innate and immutable sameness was necessary, it was an insufficient condition for entrenching race-based distinctions in the popular collective consciousness.[53] For racial classification

52 Consider one recent abstract for a report on the outcome of a research project that not only conflates the terms 'ethnicity' and 'race' but includes 'Hispanic' as one of four racial categories: 'Although osteoporosis is a worldwide health problem, there are many differences in *ethnic* groups regarding disease morbidity and drug treatment efficacy. This review analyzed clinical response data of two major osteoporotic treatments (vitamin D and estrogens) regarding *four major human races* (*Asian, Caucasian, Hispanic and Negroid*)'; F. Massart, 'Human races and pharmacogenomics of effective bone treatments', *Gynecol Endocrinol*, vol. 20, no. 1, January 2005, 36–44 (emphasis added).

53 See Ian Haney-López, *White by Law: The Legal Construction of Race* (New York: New York University Press 1996) on the terminological confusion that figured in two 1922 US Supreme Court appeal decisions for naturalization. Takao Ozawa, a Japanese applicant, successfully appealed, on scientific grounds, that he had white skin but was rejected as not being 'Caucasian' and therefore not 'white'. Three months later, Bhagat Singh Thind, a Hindu Asian petitioned for citizenship and, taking his cue from the earlier decision, argued that, according to science, Hindu Indians were of the 'Aryan' or 'Caucasian' race and, therefore, 'white'. The same judge who relied on science in his ruling in the Ozawa case, rejected Thind's claim on the basis of common sense.

to fossilize in the public consciousness as meaningful distinctions that appear *natural*, laws were needed to buttress economic and political policies of differentiation. These regulatory measures prescribed and were reinforced by everyday social norms and practices that cumulatively served to define experience. Accordingly, experience, a visceral and material way of being in the world, manifested itself as evidence for the credibility of racial distinction based on biological differences.

Given this history, one has to wonder about the cultural consensus that has come to *imagine* and *market* images that, until very recently, have excluded black and brown women from considerations of osteoporosis, a medical disease that affects post-menopausal women. Do black and brown women not suffer from osteoporosis? Or has the foundational premise of race-based categories, with *external* physiological features as the gross criteria for distinction, already prescribed answers to research questions that confirm the criteria used for race-based distinctions at the outset of the investigation? Fortunately, the Osteoporosis Center of Atlanta decided to study African-American women, a group that is 'underdiagnosed and undertreated', concluding that 'African-American and white women share many of the same risk factors for osteoporosis'.[54] Unfortunately, there are no criteria for distinguishing 'African-American' and 'white' women, who are compared as discrete *racial* units.

Genetic signature and the biologization of identity

Research on the Lemba, a group in southern Africa whose claims to Jewishness made headlines when DNA tests on their priests correlated with DNA found in Jews who were identified as *kohanim* (priests), is the most salient example of spurious claims for the utility of the race concept. The phenomenon of Jewish collective identity—despite expulsion and exile, persecution and intermarriage—refuses social science categories and taxonomy. Jews are an efficacious proxy and model for all social groups discerned as *racialized objects* by the scientific gaze. Identifying individuals as 'Jews', on the basis of purported biological criteria (DNA), is always—and in-herently—a sociological process in which biology provides false evidence of identity.[55]

According to normative rabbinical law, descent and conversion are two routes to being counted as Jewish. This rebuts claims that Jewish ancestry is revealed in a tidy *genetic signature*, a metaphor in scientific texts that anchors culturally grounded social formations to a biological foundation. When

54 Grattan C. Woodson, 'Risk factors for osteoporosis in postmenopausal African-American women', *Current Medical Research and Opinion*, vol. 20, no. 10, October 2004, 1681–7 (1686).
55 Sander L. Gilman, *The Jew's Body* (New York and London: Routledge 1991).

articles about genes and Jewish identity deploy this literary trope, the correlation between the biological existence and the social existence of Jews is made to seem natural, obfuscating the history of Jewish dispersal and diversity. Against the hope of black Americans that DNA will fill the gaps in family histories caused by slavery,[56] what purpose is served by efforts to isolate a *Jewish* gene, particularly when it is nicknamed the 'Cohen gene'?[57]

Despite frequent pronouncements that there are no biological races, the precondition for conceptualizing 'a Cohen gene' involves the preliminary assumption that evidence for a common ancestry can be found.[58] This presupposition, that the biblical Hebrews were once a distinct and discrete group, ignores the explicit ways in which the story of creating a collective identity is woven through Jewish scripture. From both a political and a sociological perspective, the unexpected 'discovery' of a priestly gene fortuitously lent credibility to the oral traditions of geographically disparate groups whose claims to Jewish identity had been ignored or dismissed as preposterous. In fact, discovery that the Y chromosome may be evidence of Jewish ancestry reignited interest in the mystery of the Lost Tribes, and focused attention on 'exotic' communities who claimed and desired a connection with world Jewry.[59]

The premise of an identifiable Jewish gene, however, is not self-evident although it offers biological credibility to myths that enable collective identities. In other words, communities grounded in a shared (even when contested) identity are above all products of sociology, not of biology. For this reason, typologies framing genetic studies of male descendants of Moses and Aaron should not be used as evidence for the continuity of stable communities. Moreover, given the rapid evolution of biotechnology,

56 Writing in the *New York Times* last summer, Amy Harmon reported: 'Some African-Americans, more interested in searching out recent relatives who in many cases can be dependably identified with a DNA match, are asking whites whom they have long suspected are cousins to take a DNA test. And in a genetic bingo game that is delivering increasing returns as people of all ethnicities engage in DNA genealogy, some are typing their results into public databases on the Internet and finding a match that no paper trail would have revealed'. Amy Harmon, 'Blacks pin hope on DNA to fill slavery's gaps in family trees', *New York Times*, 25 July 2005.

57 The 'Cohen modal haplotype' (CMH) was 'discovered' among some members of the Buba, the Lemba's senior clan somewhat analogous to the *kohen* (or Cohen) priestly clan. The sensational news of a genetic connection to Jewish ancestry was augmented as much by the fact that the Lemba are black Africans as by the lack of any reference to them in literature in any field. Mark G. Thomas, Tudor Parfitt, Deborah A. Weiss, Karl Skorecki, James F. Wilson, Magdel le Roux, Neil Bradman and David B. Goldstein, 'Y chromosomes traveling south: the Cohen modal haplotype and the origins of the Lemba—the "black Jews of Southern Africa"', *American Journal of Human Genetics*, vol. 66, no. 2, February 2000, 674–86.

58 Avshalom Zoosmann-Diskin, 'Are today's Jewish priests descended from the old ones?', *Homo: Journal of Comparative Human Biology*, vol. 51, nos 2–3, 2000, 156–62.

59 Hillel Halkin, 'Wandering Jews—and their genes', *Commentary*, vol. 110, no. 2, September 2000, 54–61.

researchers who increase their pool of subjects may find additional groups of men—who neither identify as nor are identified as Jewish or a *kohen*—who test positive for the same Y chromosome that currently appears among a select, self- and otherwise identified group with priestly lineages.[60]

The impulse to find a shared Y chromosome indicating a direct patrilineal line to Moses and Aaron seems to have inhibited less sensational investigations into the relationship between an apparent genetic signature and demographic movement in general. Issues raised by DNA sequencing invite compelling discussions about the social world in which political questions and policies occupy a central role in shaping identities and life experiences. Despite disclaimers to the contrary, announcements that particular DNA sequences indicate genetic correlation between various population groups appeal to the notion of biological race. The presumption of particular ancestral connections orients how DNA is invoked in discussions of collective identity, in which the vocabulary of genes displaces earlier metaphors of blood. The politicized relationship between science and identity is explicit when genetic research supplements, and insures a surrogate role for, cultural anthropological and archaeological evidence. For those with contested claims to Jewish identity, data presented in the specialized language of science can be authoritatively introduced as evidence for their connection with, and perhaps membership in, the Jewish diaspora, despite their distance from the geographical scope of rabbinical authorities. But if science can be invoked as a guarantor of identities, it can equally intercede to deny them.

The presumption that scientific conclusions are based on objective facts obscures the less rigorous process by which cultural interpretations of selective data are (re)presented as fact, whether it is in order to prove the utility of 'race' as an organizing concept or to argue for 'ethnicity' as a more

---

60 Judiciously, in this context, the authority of science was invoked to silence sceptics of the Lemba's claims to Jewish ancestry although it also invited speculation on whether the Lemba qualified for immediate Israeli citizenship under the Law of Return. Carl Elliott and Paul Brodwin, 'Identity and genetic ancestry tracing', *British Medical Journal*, vol. 325, 21 December 2002, 1469–71; Paul Brodwin, 'Genetics, identity and the anthropology of essentialism', *Anthropological Quarterly*, vol. 75, no. 2, Spring 2002, 323–30. Most significantly, *the manner* in which the issue of the Lemba was articulated introduced a political dimension that necessarily, given the politics of race and racism in the United States, insinuated and instantiated a racial inflection, such as in newspaper headlines like 'DNA Backs South African Tribe's Tradition of Early Descent from the Jews', 'The Black Jews of Southern Africa' and 'Jewish Roots in Africa'. Perhaps because the information was less sensational, the popular media were silent on the absence of evidence for a *kohen* genetic variant among the Jews of Ethiopia. M. F. Hammer, A. J. Redd, E. T. Wood, M. R. Bonner, H. Jarjanazi, T. Karafet, S. Santachiara-Benerecetti, A. Oppenheim, M. A. Jobling, T. Jenkins, H. Ostrer and B. Bonné-Tamir, 'Jewish and Middle Eastern non-Jewish populations share a common pool of Y-chromosome biallelic haplotypes', *Proceedings of the National Academy of Sciences*, vol. 97, no. 12, 6 June 2000, 6769–74.

efficient one. As long as human beings are categorized, classified or grouped according to preconceived ideas of similarity, racialized truths will continue to be reinscribed in research projects. In this context, the language of *genetic signature* (as in the 'CMH') is politically provocative, and scientists need to be especially conscious of the metaphors they invent to articulate the results of their research and should take serious note of Nancy Stepan's studies on the central role metaphors play in scientific theory, including the analogies they mediate.[61] In sum, the deliberate attempt to identify a shared chromosome among different populations is not an innocent pursuit that can be interpreted outside the politics of identity.[62] For this reason, academics and lay people—those with and without expertise in genetic studies—need to be vigilant in challenging the incorporation of a discourse of genes into the sociological discourse of group identities.

Letting go of race

Scientists who look to the human body to reveal itself seem unable or unwilling to relinquish the promise of guarantees that affirm essential differences as an explanation for perceived variations distinguishing communities and individuals. The hyper-visibility of the physical body (skin colour, hair texture, facial features) still attracts debate over the merit of traditional racial categories as a point of departure for research on populations. This epidermal surface, distinguishing social groups, is invested with meanings and experiences that reinforce ideas of race based on appearance.

Public pronouncements disseminating the fact that 'race' is a bogus concept are refuted by reports in science journals, forensic commentaries, newspaper headlines and pharmaceutical advertisements alleging genetic predispositions of named population groups distinguished by physical appearance and geography. Bioethicists and geneticists have now joined anthropologists, and, notwithstanding protestations to the contrary, the points of departure in their complimentary and complementary research projects prescribe outcomes that reinstate racial boundaries in thinking about ancestry, genealogy and identity.

The tendency to cluster people in familiar ways repackages racial differences under the label of variation. Finding new names for old

---

61 Nancy Leys Stepan, 'Race and gender: the role of analogy in science', in Sandra Harding (ed.), *The 'Racial' Economy of Science: Toward A Democratic Future* (Bloomington: Indiana University Press 1993), 359–76.

62 Precisely for this reason, genes are irrelevant to *religious* deliberations on the question of who is a Jew although they may be invoked in appeals for state recognition and immediate Israeli citizenship under the Law of Return.

configurations does not allow for radically different ways to cluster populations as subjects of study. I am not arguing against genetic studies *per se*, nor do I deny that deciphering genetic patterns may constructively contribute to medical research devoted to the eradication of medical disorders, disease and chronic illnesses. But it cannot be over-emphasized that the social categories that scientists have been using are permeable and flexible. While they are instructive when examining the socio-political ways in which people identify themselves and are identified, a radical cultural shift is needed.

As the sociologist Paul Gilroy observes: 'Whether it is articulated in the more specialized tongues of biological science and pseudo-science, or in a vernacular idiom of culture and common sense, the term "race" conjures up a peculiarly resistant variety of natural difference.'[63] We need to ask what difference does difference make? What cultural predispositions inform scholarly research that takes human variability as its focal point? And we need accountability on the part of both researchers and their funding agencies, who should address the question of why it is important to find a genetic code. For whom is the enormous investment in time, energy and capital of significance? Most importantly, why does determining biological difference take priority over variations in the quality of life among humankind? Given the racial context that frames genetic research by default—if not intent—Gilroy's compelling appeal for liberation from 'all racializing and raciological thought, from racialized seeing, racialized thinking and racialized thinking about thinking' as 'the only ethical response to the conspicuous wrongs that raciologies continue to solicit and sanction' needs to be broadcast far and wide and heeded throughout the field(s) of bio-science.[64]

Katya Gibel Azoulay is Associate Professor of Anthropology and American Studies at Grinnell College, Iowa. She is the author of *Black, Jewish and Interracial: It's Not the Color of Your Skin but the Race of Your Kin and Other Myths of Identity* (Duke University Press 1997).

63 Paul Gilroy, *Against Race: Imagining Political Culture beyond the Color Line* (Cambridge, MA: Belknap Press of the Harvard University Press 2000), 29.
64 Ibid., 40–1.

Folk taxonomy, prejudice and the human genome: using disease as a Jewish ethnic marker

JUDITH S. NEULANDER

ABSTRACT   When the Human Genome Project was completed, scientists discovered whole new populations that were at risk of heritable disorders. This revelation entails an obligation to be scientifically accurate and socially responsible in the biological classification, or labelling, of these populations. Neulander will define as unscientific 'folk taxonomy' all biological classification according to cultural commonalities: those traits and characteristics that—like religious affiliation—can only be acquired through learning, and are not biologically heritable. Noting the widespread popularity of sweeping cultural characteristics into biological classification—as in use of the term 'Jewish' for certain heritable diseases—she examines the social consequences of giving religious labels to genetic disorders in multiracial New Mexico, where disease-based claims of 'secret' or crypto-Jewish forebears are being used to assert an overvalued line of white ancestral descent, and where use of the term 'Jewish' to determine who is at risk of heritable diseases is generating, in turn, the use of heritable diseases to determine who is a Jew. The phenomenon will be examined in both folkloric and academic contexts, since locals who seek crypto-Jewish legitimacy thereby striate, into colour-coded levels of human valuation, what is otherwise a cohesive society, bringing their academic enablers into active, legitimating complicity. Neulander's essay seeks to help readers distinguish between folkloric and academic motivations and methods for discerning and describing human differences. Finally, she proposes a more valid and reliable means of classifying populations at risk of heritable disorders, the better to ensure results that are both scientifically accurate and socially responsible.

> *The Ariadne thread in botany is classification, without which there is chaos.*
> —Carl Linnaeus (1707–78)

Efforts to map the human genome require modern taxonomists to define new, and sometimes unanticipated, categories of human variation. But human differences—biological or otherwise—have never been easy to define. Even Linnaeus, master taxonomist and father of modern scientific classification, dropped Ariadne's thread when he entered the maze of human distinctions. Drawing biological boundaries around the cultural characteristics of indigenous peoples, he constructed inaccurate, over-inclusive folk categories and, in so doing, reinforced a self-authenticating colonial world-view that justified savagery in the name of civilization. This is not because Linnaeus was an ill-intentioned or inferior scientist. Rather, despite good character and strong intellect, he was a product of his own cultural milieu, and his culturally determined knowledge—like our own —was so deeply entrenched as 'the way things are', he was unable to grasp its arbitrary nature. It follows that, faced with the task of defining newly discovered genetic populations—how to classify different groups at risk of heritable diseases, for example—some of our modern, analytical categories may be nothing more than folk taxonomies in disguise.[1]

To help avoid a modern recycling of colonial folk taxonomy, this essay will distinguish academic logic from folk logic in the context of the human genome. As an example of a modern, genomic folk taxonomy, we will examine New Mexican use of ailments labelled 'Jewish' to classify Spanish Americans as descendants of Jews. As we are about to see, claims of Judaeo-Spanish ancestry are used to assert an overvalued line of white ancestral descent in the American Southwest: a phenotypical line of ancestry regionally assumed for all Jews, but not for all Spanish Americans. Hence, use of a 'Jewish' label for ailments found, or imagined, among Spanish Americans of New Mexico, both reflects and reinforces a regional scale of human valuation, striating into colour-coded degrees of human degradation what is otherwise a socially cohesive community. We will therefore consider an alternative to the use of religious labels for heritable diseases, since it is precisely this academic practice that enables and legitimates the popular recycling of colonial folk taxonomies, like the one that persists in New Mexico.

In defining categories of human variation, the distinction between academic logic and folk logic is straightforward. Academic logic discerns categories by differential, critical thinking; it strives for timeless, global accuracy, no matter what may be discovered. Folk logic, however, has a different purpose than accuracy. To paraphrase Hayden White, folk categories of human distinction are self-authenticating social devices, involving not merely the clarity, but also the self-esteem and perceived entitlements of the group doing the categorizing.[2] As folklorist Dan Ben-Amos puts it:

> Analytical [academic] categories ... have been developed in the context of scholarship and serve its varied research purposes. Native [folk] taxonomy, on the other hand, has no external objective. The logical principles that underlie its

1 Alan Dundes, 'The number three in American culture', in Alan Dundes (ed.), *Interpreting Folklore* (Bloomington: Indiana University Press 1980), 134–59 (155).
2 Hayden White, *The Tropics of Discourse: Essays in Cultural Criticism* (Baltimore and London: Johns Hopkins University Press 1985), 151.

categorization ... are those which are meaningful to the members of the group and can guide them in their personal relationships.[3]

We over-generalize, or create over-inclusive folk categories, when we identify genetically linked populations the same way Linnaeus did: according to non-heritable factors, namely, those particular traits and characteristics (like religious affiliation) that can only be acquired through learning, that may exist only in the eye of the beholder, or—as applies specifically to religion—that involve 'volatile, inward states known subjectively, if at all'.[4] Clearly, the extent, and even the reality, of a group's non-heritable traits and characteristics are at best unstable, if not entirely uncertain, making them essentially untestable. Thus, a heritable disease originating in a geographical area like West Africa will correlate more accurately to persons with ancestral origins in that area than to arbitrary religious categories like 'Christians' or 'Protestants'. Similarly, populations carrying a heritable disease from a French Canadian founder will correlate more accurately to persons of French Canadian descent than to the category 'Catholics', even though most descendants may be Catholic and may no longer live in Canada. It follows that populations carrying a heritable disease from an Eastern European founder will correlate more accurately to persons of Eastern European descent than to the category 'Jews'. But we are conditioned to dispute the last instance, for the category 'Jew' is by definition over-inclusive in our culture, given the widespread Euro-American failure to differentiate between heritable characteristics acquired only through DNA and the cultural characteristics widely attributed to Jews, some of which are wholly imagined and the rest of which are acquired only by learning. Our societal propensity for over-generalization of Cultural Others is hardly limited to Jews, but, as Gordon W. Allport writes:

> The most clear of all is the case of the Jews. While they are primarily a religious group, they are likewise viewed as a race, a nation, a people, a culture. When religious distinctions are made to do double duty, the grounds for prejudice are laid, for prejudice means that inept, over-inclusive categories are employed in place of differential thinking.[5]

---

3 Dan Ben-Amos, 'Analytic categories and ethnic genres', in Dan Ben-Amos (ed.), *Folklore Genres* (Austin and London: University of Texas Press 1976), 215–42 (225).

4 Roy A. Rapapport, 'Ritual', in Richard Bauman (ed.), *Folklore, Cultural Performances and Popular Entertainments: A Communications-Centered Handbook* (New York and Oxford: Oxford University Press 1992), 253.

5 Gordon W. Allport, *The Nature of Prejudice*, 25th Anniversary edn (Reading, MA: Addison-Wesley Publishing Company 1994), 446.

The 'discovery' of New Mexican crypto-Jews

For a modern instance of genetic over-generalization, involving Jews as well as prejudice, we turn first to the state of New Mexico in the mid-1970s, when longstanding Spanish-American claims of descent from Spanish conquistadors were fully discredited.[6] Regional claims of a prestigious aristocratic (ostensibly monogamous and white) lineage date back to at least the founding of modern New Mexico at the turn of the eighteenth century. By that time the Spanish-American population included African and American Indian admixture, a profile so undervalued by the founding fathers that they institutionalized what Chilean sociologist Alejandro Lipschutz calls a 'pigmentocracy',[7] a formal caste system based on skin colour and phenotype, which in New Mexico was calculated in twenty-two degrees of increasing distance from the ideal of unbroken white European descent.[8] As Ramón Gutiérrez writes of Spain and New Mexico:

> The whiter one's skin, the greater one's claim to the honor and precedence Spaniards expected and received. The darker a person's skin, the closer one was presumed to be to the physical labor of slaves and tributary Indians, and the closer the visual association with the infamy of the conquered. In Spain families guarded their *limpieza de sangre* or blood purity through avoidance of Moors and Jews. In New Mexico, families of aristocratic pretension feared that their bloodlines might be metaphysically polluted by Indians, *mulatos*, and as one man put it, 'castes which are held or reputed as despicable in this kingdom.'[9]

Spanish Jews were undoubtedly among those ranked despicable on the Spanish colonial social scale. So much so that their exclusion from the brutally ostracizing New Mexican caste system is a powerful indicator that none were there to be brutally ostracized. Rather, reflecting the popular colonial conflation of indigenous peoples with the 'lost tribes' of Israel,

6 Nancie L. González, *The Spanish-Americans of New Mexico: A Heritage of Pride* (Albuquerque: University of New Mexico Press 1969), 81; Fr Angelico Chávez, *Origins of New Mexican Families in the Spanish Colonial Period, in Two Parts: The Seventeenth (1598–1693) and the Eighteenth (1693–1821) Centuries* (Santa Fe, NM: William Gannon 1975), xiv, xvi.
7 Alejandro Lipschutz, *El indoamericanismo y el problema racial en las Americas* (Santiago: Nascimento 1944), 75.
8 Ramón A. Gutiérrez, *When Jesus Came the Corn Mothers Went Away: Marriage, Sexuality and Power in New Mexico, 1500–1846* (Stanford, CA: Stanford University Press 1991), 198; Pedro Alonso O'Crouley, *A Description of the Kingdom of New Spain* [1744], trans. from the Spanish by Seán Galvin (San Francisco: John Howell 1972), 19; Adrian H. Bustamante, 'Españoles, castas y labradores: Santa Fe society in the eighteenth century', in David Grant Noble (ed.), *Santa Fe: History of an Ancient City* (Santa Fe, NM: School of American Research Press 1989), 64–77, *passim*.
9 Gutiérrez, *When Jesus Came the Corn Mothers Went Away*, 198–9.

Alejandro Mora, a resident of Bernalillo in 1751, gave what was then a socially acceptable explanation for beating an Indian slave: "'God has given me life," said Mora, "so that I might do to these Jews what they did to our Holiest Lord".'[10] But, by 1975, when Spanish-American claims of aristocratic white descent were finally discredited, the notion of unbroken descent from (ostensibly monogamous and white) Jews, who introduced ostensibly tell-tale folkways into the region, became the best, and perhaps last, means of denying non-white admixture and restoring the local prestige lineage. Thus, almost immediately, ambiguously Jewish artefacts introduced by early twentieth-century Adventist, Apostolic or 'messianic' Protestant experimentation (such as six-pointed stars on cemetery crosses, abstention from pork, Saturday observance of the Sabbath, giving Old Testament names to children etc.) were taken for, and touted as, evidence of Judaeo-Spanish, or colonial 'Sephardi', descent.[11]

Upon careful investigation, there is no evidence from the past nor anything visible in the present to indicate Sephardi descent for the founding fathers of Spanish New Mexico. Rather, the documented historical and cultural records refute any such claim.[12] For an objective research project that draws conclusions based on relevant genetic data, readers should see the study by Wesley Sutton et al. at Stanford University.[13] This study found that, for all relevant Y chromosome markers, paternal ancestry of New Mexican Spanish Americans is identical (except for 2.2 per cent American Indian admixture) to that observed in modern, post-exilic Spain, and is significantly different from all Jewish populations, including Iberian Jews. Had crypto-Jewish claims been accurate, there would be a higher rate of Iberian Jewish ancestry in New Mexico, reflecting a component of exiled Iberian Jews among the region's Spanish settlers. But the evidence from New Mexican Spanish-American males is unequivocal: regional claims of crypto-Jewish descent are refuted by the genetic profile of this population. Nevertheless, there is a historical and cultural precedent for claiming Judaeo-Spanish descent throughout the Spanish Americas. As

10 Ibid., 195.
11 Judith S. Neulander, 'The New Mexican crypto-Jewish canon: choosing to be "chosen" in millennial tradition', Jewish Folklore and Ethnology Review, vol. 18, nos 1–2, 1996, 19–58; Judith S. Neulander, 'Cannibals, Castes and Crypto-Jews: Premillennial Cosmology in Post Colonial New Mexico', Ph.D. dissertation, Indiana University, 2001; Judith S. Neulander, 'Jews, Crypto-', in Simon J. Bronner (ed.), Encyclopedia of American Folklife, 4 vols (Armonk, NY: M. E. Sharpe 2006).
12 Neulander, 'The New Mexican crypto-Jewish canon'.
13 Wesley K. Sutton, Alec Knight, Peter A. Underhill, Judith S. Neulander, Todd R. Disotell and Joanna L. Mountain, 'Toward resolution of the debate regarding purported crypto-Jews in a Spanish-American population: evidence from the Y-chromosome', Annals of Human Biology, vol. 33, no. 1, January–February 2006, 100–11.

Raphael Patai wrote on the phenomenon of Spanish-American identity-switching:

> To trace one's ancestry to Spain has meant to establish a claim to high status, to a prestige lineage. It is a frequent phenomenon for an Indian to claim to be a mestizo [of mixed blood] and for a mestizo to claim pure Spanish descent ... Spanish descent, even Spanish-Jewish descent, means a step up on the social scale.[14]

Hence, in 1980, New Mexico hired as its new State Historian Stanley M. Hordes, who had written a doctoral dissertation on secretly professing or 'crypto-Jews' in the Spanish Americas. His arrival provoked a spate of rumours, gossip and hearsay concerning ambiguously Jewish (and, there-fore, ostensibly white) regional folkways. Hordes announced to the press and media that a significant component of 'crypto-Jews' were indeed among the region's early Spanish settlers, the Jewish origin of their folkways having been effectively forgotten.[15] Shortly thereafter, a small but vocal group of Spanish Americans, their memories thus 'restored', came forward to claim publicly their new prestige lineage. Undeterred by the indisputably Portuguese origin of colonial America's crypto-Jews,[16] or by the indisputably Spanish origin of modern New Mexico's founding fathers,[17] a similarly small and vocal number of academics—none of whom was a folklore specialist—also came forward to endorse New Mexico's modern, and primarily Protestant, folkways as both colonial and crypto-Jewish.

At this point, the use of heritable disease as a marker for Jewish descent was a topic of local gossip, but no purported instance was recorded in print. That would occur more than a decade later, after all folkloric evidence of New Mexican crypto-Jewish descent had been discredited by my detailed criticism of New Mexican claims, published in 1996.[18] In response, creators and promoters of the popular canon began to seek a legitimating 'scientific' means to strengthen their claims. To popular, pseudo-ethnographic con-structions of New Mexican Sephardi folkways they added popular, pseudo-scientific constructions of New Mexican Sephardi diseases. In this way, academic use of the label 'Jewish' to determine who is at risk of heritable

14 Raphael Patai, 'The Jewish Indians of Mexico', in R. Patai, *On Jewish Folklore* (Detroit: Wayne State University Press 1983), 447–75 (461).
15 Stanley M. Hordes, 'The Sephardic legacy in the Southwest: crypto-Jews of New Mexico, historical research project sponsored by the Latin American Institute, University of New Mexico', *Jewish Folklore and Ethnology Review*, vol. 15, no. 2, 1993, 137–8.
16 Seymour B. Liebman, *The Inquisitors and the Jews in the New World: Summaries of Procesos, 1500–1810, and Bibliographic Guide* (Coral Gables, FL: University of Miami Press 1974).
17 Chávez, *Origins of New Mexican Families in the Spanish Colonial Period*.
18 Neulander, 'The New Mexican crypto-Jewish canon'.

diseases paved the way for popular use of heritable diseases to determine who is a Jew.

Accordingly, criticism is due Kristine Bordenave, a dermatologist who conducted a study meant to use pemphigus vulgaris (PV), a globally distributed, autoimmune blister rash, as a Jewish ethnic marker in New Mexico.[19] Bordenave concluded that the high incidence of PV among New Mexican Spanish Americans indicated their descent from Jews, since Jews have a similarly high incidence of PV. The space allotted here will not suffice to criticize the undifferentiated, over-inclusive conflation of Spanish-speaking and Jewish populations required to support Bordenave's conclusion. Suffice it to say that a full year before a reprise of her study was published in Hordes's recent book,[20] Ron Loewenthal and his colleagues found that disease haplotypes for PV are neither of ancient nor of Middle Eastern origin, but are relatively recent and originate with a Mediterranean forebear.[21] Regarding Spaniards and Jews, the Loewenthal *et al.* study found that the 'distance between the two PV cohorts is relatively short, but the distance between Jewish patients and Jewish controls is greater compared to the distance between Spanish patients and Spanish controls'.[22] Hence, the ancestral condition appears to have occurred first in Spaniards and then spread to Jewish populations. Moreover, as Sutton *et al.* showed in 2006, the paternal profile of New Mexican Spanish Americans is highly significantly different from that of all Jews, including Iberian Jews, and at the same time is indistinguishable from Mediterranean Spaniards (except for 2.2 per cent American Indian admixture).[23] Therefore, the more logical conclusion is that high incidence of PV among New Mexican Spanish Americans does not indicate descent from Jews, but reflects instead descent from the same Mediterranean forebears who spread PV to Jews.

19 Kristine K. Bordenave, Jeffrey Griffith, Stanley M. Hordes, Thomas M. Williams and R. Steven Padilla, 'The historical and geomedical immunogenetics of pemphigus among the descendants of Sephardic Jews in New Mexico', *Archives of Dermatology*, vol. 137, no. 6, June 2001, 825–6.

20 Kristine Bordenave and Stanley M. Hordes, 'Pemphigus vulgaris among Hispanos in New Mexico and its possible connection with crypto-Jewish populations', in Stanley M. Hordes, *To the End of the Earth: A History of the Crypto-Jews of New Mexico* (New York: Columbia University Press 2005), 289–95. I have been commissioned to review this book by several journals, including *Shofar*, the *Catholic Historical Review* and the *Journal of American Folklore*; the reviews will appear in late 2006 or early in 2007.

21 Ron Loewenthal, Yelena Slomov, Maria Francisca Gonzalez-Escribano, Ilan Goldberg, Michael Korostishevsky, Sarah Brenner, A. Nuñez-Roldan, Julián Sánchez Conejo-Mir and Ephraim Gazit, 'Common ancestral origin of pemphigus vulgaris in Jews and Spaniards: a study using microsatellite markers', *Tissue Antigens*, vol. 63, no. 4, April 2004, 326–34.

22 Ibid., 326.

23 Sutton *et al.*, 'Toward resolution of the debate regarding purported crypto-Jews in a Spanish-American population'.

Constructing legends

As Mary Louise Pratt writes: 'In any global classificatory project, the observing and cataloging of evidence itself becomes narratable, able to constitute a sequence of events, or even produce a plot ... [to] form the main storyline of an entire account.'[24] It is therefore revealing that the narrative genre most often employed for reporting disease-based discoveries of crypto-Jews is a traditional folk genre, one that sometimes employs academic formats (footnotes, endnotes etc.), but never reflects academic substance. Such narratives are typically built on urban legends: tales that circulate outward from modern urban centres, typically reflecting local preoccupations and social agendas.

In New Mexico, for example, typical reports of surviving crypto-Jewish customs are described as having been reported to, rather than witnessed by, the person telling us about them. This subtype of legend, from which we never get first-hand or eyewitness information, is classified as a *FOAFtale* in folkloristic scholarship. The acronym stands for 'Friend-of-a-Friend', since the primary source of information in such tales (the friend of a friend, or the friend's friend of a friend ... etc.) is always anonymous or too far removed to secure or verify the claims being made.

Unlike myths (which fill lacunae in time beyond recall when world and social order were still being formed), and unlike fairytales (which take place in formulaic time, like 'once upon a time' and 'happily ever after'), legends always take place in historical time. Thus, a legend is a story involving a historical person, place or event, but is about something that cannot be secured or verified in history (e.g. an influx of crypto-Jews into colonial New Mexico or sightings of Elvis along the nation's highways). Legends therefore gain credibility through a compelling combination of superficial plausibility and popular appeal. Relying on our propensity to lend credibility to any intrinsically satisfying or otherwise appealing plausibility, legends are always told as true stories.[25]

Thus it was in Santa Fe, in the summer of 1992, when Hordes mentioned to me that he was looking into a disease called 'Niemann-Pick' as confirmation of Spanish-American descent from crypto-Jews. This may not be the first attempt to use heritable disease as a Jewish ethnic marker in New Mexico, but it was the first time I had heard the proposition. The conversation would gain greater folkloristic significance six months later, in a coffee house in Albuquerque, when a young man clearly convinced of his crypto-Jewish origin, informed me that 'a rabbi in Colorado' had

24 Mary Louise Pratt, *Imperial Eyes: Travel Writing and Transculturation* (London and New York: Routledge 1992), 27–8.
25 Alan Dundes, 'Madness and method plus a plea for protective inversion in myth', in Laurie L. Patton and Wendy Doniger (eds), *Myth and Method* (Charlottesville and London: University Press of Virginia 1996), 147–59 (147).

recognized a Spanish-American woman to be Jewish based on her mother's affliction with a 'Jewish' disease. I could not determine whether the tale came first, and had inspired Hordes's interest in disease-based Judaism, or whether Hordes's interest had come first, generating a self-authenticating tale of disease-based Judaism among would-be descendants of crypto-Jews. But, as we are about to see, the publication of this tale ten years later, as narrated by an anonymous source claiming to be the woman whose mother had the 'Jewish' disease, confirms its ongoing circulation in local oral tradition. By the same token, the publication of this account by an academic, Janet Liebman Jacobs, constitutes yet another telling: one embellished by academic commentary, and endorsed as 'history' by virtue of the authority vested in a university press.[26]

However, had I not heard a variant of the same tale ten years earlier, the repetitions would still allow us to identify the story as a folk narrative, according to Stith Thompson, the grand old man of folktale classification. Thompson defines as a folk 'motif' the smallest element of any tale that is striking or unusual;[27] thus, 'mother' is not a folk motif, but 'wicked stepmother' is. As Thompson notes, the narration of any striking or unusual element, more than once, not only classifies it as a motif, but also indicates its 'power to persist in tradition', adding that striking or unusual *incidents* comprise the vast majority of folk motifs that represent a category of tale, or tale-type.[28] When an unusual incident is (or can be) secured and verified, we automatically classify it as 'history'. But as long as an unusual incident remains unsecured and unverified, no one representing academe is at liberty to misrepresent it as a historical event (even if it reportedly occurred in a particular location and at a specified time). Thus, the unusual 'rabbi in Colorado' incident, which has remained unsecured and unverified for more than ten years, is by definition not history. It persists only as an unsecured, unverified narrative, therefore as a legend, and one that is destined to remain so by virtue of its *FOAFtale* format.

Although we could easily call this narrative the 'rabbi in Colorado' story, there is nothing striking or unusual about a rabbi being in Colorado, in and of itself. Therefore, folkloristic analysis requires parsing the motif—the striking or unusual incident itself—for productive study, in this case, for example: 'individual's hidden identity revealed to an authenticating pundit through relative's heritable disease'. Parsing the unusual incident in this minimalist way allows a given variant to be discerned from other possible variants within the tale-type, each according to its own regional or ethnic specificity. In this case, the Southwestern Spanish-American variant would

26 Janet Liebman Jacobs, *Hidden Heritage: The Legacy of the Crypto-Jews* (Berkeley and Los Angeles: University of California Press 2002).
27 Stith Thompson, *The Folktale* (Los Angeles: University of California Press 1977), 114.
28 Ibid., 115.

be: 'Spanish-American daughter's hidden Jewish identity revealed to Colorado rabbi through mother's heritable Niemann-Pick disease.'

For any folk narrative to persist, however, it must contain a number of negotiable traits: elements that can be modified without changing what the tale is about. This enables the tale to dodge later discreditation, to take on other ethnic identities and/or to enhance its literary impact. Such negotiable traits include names and ages of protagonists, genders, national identities and religious affiliations, and—as would occur in the case of the Niemann-Pick tale—the name of the disease in question. The reason for this latter modification is worth noting, since it does not reflect a change in the spirit or mentality of crypto-Jewish reporting in modern New Mexico.

Jewish by disease

According to the medical literature, the term 'Niemann-Pick' refers to a group of 'storage' disorders in which waste materials build up in human tissue and cause it to deteriorate. Since storage disorders are found among Jews, and also among Spanish Americans of New Mexico (as well as in other populations), the introduction of Niemann-Pick allows for the superficial plausibility of a genetic link between Spanish Jews and Spanish Americans. But in over-inclusive folk logic, the discovery of any plausibility constitutes its full confirmation. Hence, the activity recognized as 'research' by academics—the critical, differential logic required to confirm or deny a given plausibility—is never undertaken. Not surprisingly, even the most rudimentary investigation reveals that Niemann-Pick types A and B, alone, are found among Jews, but only among Ashkenazi (Germanic) Jews. Clearly, a disease not known to occur among Sephardi (Iberian) Jews cannot be used as an ethnic marker for Sephardi descent, as it is in the New Mexican tale of Niemann-Pick. With regard to the Spanish-American population, the tale similarly fails to differentiate Niemann-Pick types A and B from Niemann-Pick type C, which is the only type found among Spanish Americans of New Mexico and is a different disease at both the biochemical and genetic level.[29] Thus, the tale could only retain Niemann-Pick as long as the flaw in its logic went unrecognized. At some point the disease would have to change if the tale was to retain even superficial plausibility.

It was roughly six years after the folkloristic discreditation of 1996 that the crypto-Jewish canon in general, and a variant of the Niemann-Pick legend in particular, first gained academic legitimacy through a university press.[30] In Liebman Jacobs's work on New Mexican folkways, we find the only printed version of the Niemann-Pick legend. Told as a true story, the text retains the

29 Laith F. Gulli and Tanya Bivins, 'Niemann-Pick disease', in Stacey L. Blachford (ed.), *The Gale Encyclopedia of Genetic Disorders*, 2 vols (Detroit: Gale Group 2002), ii.813–16.
30 Liebman Jacobs, *Hidden Heritage*.

daughter with the hidden identity, the rabbi in Colorado and the afflicted mother, but it replaces Niemann-Pick with Creutzfeldt-Jakob Disease (CJD). The substitute illness, known as heritable or 'familial' CJD, is an extremely rare, degenerative disease with a well documented and unusually high incidence among Libyan Jews.[31] The substitution of CJD for Niemann-Pick therefore indicates that those who tell the tale believe Libyan Jews to be of Spanish origin, and also believe that heritable CJD has been found among Southwestern Spanish Americans, although—as we are about to see—both beliefs are incorrect. The timing of the substitution indicates that Niemann-Pick lost credibility some time after 1992, when it was first mentioned to me, and before 2002, when the CJD variant was first published. Alternatively, the substitution may simply represent a literary strategy inspired by the British 'mad cow' epidemic of the late 1990s, which—having been identified as CJD by the media—would have lent CJD greater literary impact than the similarly heritable, but less sensationalized Niemann-Pick disease.

The published narrative is important for understanding how easily an over-inclusive folk category of human genetic identity can be constructed at the academic level. As can be seen in this particular case, the academic mission need only succumb to the thrall of discovering lost/hidden Jews, thus preserving the academic format while building exclusively on classic elements of folk logic: over-generalization of superficially related parallels, facile placement of Jewish labels on persons who otherwise are not identifiable as Jews, use of pseudepigraphy (false ascription of authenticating statements to authorities who never made them), and—with regard to recognizing and interpreting folkloric material—a complete innocence (or wholesale rejection) of all theories, techniques and methods of folkloristic enquiry, classification and interpretation.

The *FOAFtale* and its commentary take up less than a single page in Liebman Jacobs's book, prefaced by a relatively long discussion of matrilineal descent as the traditional, rabbinic means of establishing one's status as a Jew. Thus, the issue of matrilineal descent serves as a distraction from the primary factor that actually impedes Spanish-American claims to Jewish descent: today's most elderly Spanish Americans (like their fathers before them) are professing Christians. This creates a problem for Spanish Americans seeking recognition as Jews, since Jewish status cannot be claimed by persons of non-Jewish descent who cannot document a personal Jewish history, and who themselves profess other religions. Hence, given the talmudic precept that descent from a Jewish mother automatically secures Jewish status, the solution for one non-Jewish individual (rendered anonymous by Liebman Jacobs) was to demonstrate the regionally coveted (white) bloodline through maternal affliction with a fancifully constructed

31 Zeev Meiner, Ruth Gabizon and Stanley B. Prusiner, 'Familial Creutzfeldt-Jakob disease: codon 200 prion disease in Libyan Jews', *Medicine* (Baltimore), vol. 76, no. 4, July 1997, 227–37.

'Sephardi' disease. Interestingly, this congenitally diseased construction of Judaism, emptied of all religious meaning, does indeed trace back to an ancestral Spanish legacy; it reflects the (obviously persistent) Spanish colonial belief that Jews do not constitute a faith community but, instead, belong to a biologically immutable 'race', unaffected by religious affiliation.[32]

As we are about to see, all scientific and religious claims made in this tale are demonstrably unfounded but, as a folktale, it has a different goal than that of accuracy; it exists to enable the Spanish-American narrator to take a desired step-up on the regional Southwestern pigmentocracy by virtue of her mother's 'Sephardi' disease, thereby compelling 'Jewish' recognition according to the same rabbinic law that otherwise impedes it. Liebman Jacobs, who frames the tale as a true story, upholds talmudic protocols regarding matrilineal descent, but subsequently falls from grace by claiming CJD as one of them, informing her readers: '... only one descendant in this study was recognized as Jewish through blood ties to the mother' (as was purportedly 'revealed' by heritable CJD).[33]

Notably, before the tale is even begun, the so-called descendant's crypto-Jewish lineage is given as rabbinically 'recognized' (albeit by an anonymous character in a narrative who himself cannot be recognized). The narrator's 'Jewish' identity is additionally confirmed by academic fiat, since the author refers to the narrator as a 'descendant', although the author herself never secured or verified the evidence given for that claim. Moreover, Liebman Jacobs follows the narrator's lead, rendering all primary sources anonymous, thereby making it virtually impossible for anyone else to secure or verify the same information. Clearly, the interview is a violation of scholarly norms, and meets no standards set by any academic discipline. It is instead a garden variety *FOAFtale* in which the author is our academic 'friend', who tells us what she heard from her Spanish-American friend (the FOAF), while the key rabbinical figure—a friend of the author's friend (who could certainly have given both women the credibility they so clearly desire)—is someone both anonymous and too far removed (living 'somewhere' in Colorado) to be reached for verification. Not surprisingly, Liebman Jacobs's preamble mis- and disinforms, biasing her readers instead of enlightening them: 'In this case the descendant's mother suffered from Creutzfeldt-Jacob [*sic*] disease, a degenerative disease of the central nervous system that has been linked specifically to Sephardic ancestry.'[34]

This statement is inaccurate on two counts. First, CJD occurs in more than one form, only one of which is heritable and, as we have seen, is found at much higher frequency among Libyan Jews than in other populations (in

---

32 Jane Berger, *The Jews of Spain: A History of the Sephardic Experience* (New York: The Free Press 1994), 127.
33 Liebman Jacobs, *Hidden Heritage*, 103.
34 Ibid.

which it also occurs). But Libyan Jews have no Sephardi connection. By the fifth century BCE Libya had a substantial Jewish population, perhaps as many as 30,000 according to the somewhat impressionistic reporting of Pliny and Herodotus.[35] Nonetheless, the Jewish population was clearly large enough to suggest tens of thousands roughly 700 years before the first artefactual evidence of a Jewish presence in Spain, in the third century CE.[36] Moreover, according to documented diasporic patterns, Libya was not among the havens sought by Spanish Jews when they left Spain in 1492; the more attractive North African destinations were Fez and Tlemcen in the nearby Barbary states, as well as Algiers, Tunisia and the city of Alexandria, then part of the Ottoman empire.[37] Hence, while there may have been the odd unrecorded instance of Spanish settlement, Libyan Jews are not a Spanish people; they have no such origin nor any subsequent history. On the other hand, while heritable CJD is well documented among them, there is no documentation of heritable CJD among descendants of Spanish Jews anywhere on the globe. Liebman Jacobs thus confirms, in a work published by a university press, that heritable CJD is a 'Sephardic' disease even though it has never been found in any Sephardi population. Furthermore, since there has also been no recorded instance of heritable CJD among Spanish Americans in the Southwest, the notion of CJD as a genetic link between Spanish Jews and Southwestern Spanish Americans lacks any credibility at all.

Second, the source used by Liebman Jacobs to link CJD with 'specifically Sephardic ancestry' is Richard M. Goodman, a recognized expert on genetic diseases found among different populations of Jews. But the article cited was published by Goodman in 1979, before any form of CJD was recognized as heritable. Hence, Liebman Jacobs resorts to pseudepigraphy, ascribing to Goodman an authenticating link—here between CJD and 'specifically Sephardic ancestry'—that he never made. Thus, we should not be surprised that Goodman, who addressed the question of heritable CJD under the heading 'Misconceptions', stated that CJD was not known to be a heritable disease: exactly the opposite of what Liebman Jacobs attributed to him. Moreover, with regard to the one Libyan outbreak known at the time, he speculated that it may have been caused by eating infected meat; a link to 'specifically Sephardic ancestry' was never mentioned, and was clearly never considered, by Goodman.[38]

35 John Wright, *Libya* (New York and Washington, D.C.: Praeger 1969), 45, 54.
36 Benjamin R. Gampel, 'Jews, Christians and Muslims in medieval Iberia: *convivencia* through the eyes of Sephardic Jews', in Vivian B. Mann, Thomas F. Glick and Jerrilyn D. Dodds (eds), *Convivencia: Jews, Muslims and Christians in Medieval Spain* (New York: George Braziller in association with the Jewish Museum 1992), 2–27 (11).
37 Gérard Chaliand and Jean-Pierre Rageau, *The Penguin Atlas of Diasporas*, trans. from the French by A. M. Berrett (New York and London: Viking Press 1995), 30–1.
38 Richard M. Goodman, *Genetic Disorders among the Jewish People* (Baltimore: Johns Hopkins University Press 1979), 409.

Thus, following a medically untrained informant instead of any easily accessible medical encyclopaedia—or even the outdated reference she cites, which also refutes her claims—Liebman Jacobs informs us that CJD is a recognized 'Sephardic' disease, and states that a Spanish-American woman's search for Jewish roots led her to 'approach a rabbi in Colorado'. On hearing that the woman's mother had CJD (in the informant's own words):

> 'The rabbi said, "You're Jewish. It doesn't make any difference if you are an atheist, you are Jewish. You don't have to convert. You can just start practicing the laws if that's what you want to do."'
>
> In recalling this aspect of her search for Jewish roots, she spoke of both the relief and sadness that accompanied her mother's diagnosis and the rabbi's affirmation of her Jewish lineage:
>
> 'It was great to find out positively that I was Jewish. I had already been researching it, so I was pretty sure that we were Jewish. So I was relieved that I didn't have to research my mother's side anymore.'[39]

Here, a modern Spanish-American *FOAFtale* attempts to authenticate religiously empty, disease-based Judaism by appeals to the two most powerfully legitimating contexts of our time: science and religion. However, as we have already seen, both science and religion negate the claims being made. Biogenetic research has unequivocally refuted any influx of exilic crypto-Jews into colonial New Mexico, and there is no CJD-Sephardi link to indicate Jewish descent through an infected mother. Moreover, according to rabbinic law, any individual professing a religion other than Judaism who seeks rabbinic recognition as a Jew must either convert or forego that recognition. Hence, we can see that this tale has a more immediate purpose than mere accuracy. It is more clearly a self-authenticating social device, meant to secure for the would-be descendant public recognition of a higher 'rank' than she could otherwise claim on the regional Spanish-American pigmentocracy: a rank she is determined to make unimpeachable in the face of any and all argument, by means of a rabbinic law on 'blood ties' to a (CJD-infected = Jewish = white) mother.

Although CJD cannot be used as a marker for Sephardi descent, we might find a way to believe this narrator if we were to assume her mother suffered from an undocumented case of heritable CJD, and she was simply misinformed by a rabbi in Colorado. In bringing the narrative to an end, however, her own testimony eliminates this possibility for, if her mother had indeed had heritable CJD, the way in which this disease is diagnosed could not possibly have escaped her:

> We knew my mother was ill. We knew she had a condition that *wasn't getting any better*. You know, it was hard knowing that my mother was ill in the first place.

39 Liebman Jacobs, *Hidden Heritage*, 103.

That was pretty tough. So the emotions were kind of mixed, because I was relieved that we were Jewish, but, you know, it's heartbreaking to see your mother go through that.[40]

The informant never pays tribute to a mother who passed away before the encounter with the rabbi. Rather, she consistently refers to a *living* mother who *wasn't getting any better* at the time of the encounter. Hence, we learn that the rabbi's recognition evoked, on the one hand, relief that the heritable disease revealed the daughter's hidden identity and, on the other, heartbreak at the sight of the mother's ongoing suffering. Yet, to date, there is only one possible way to diagnose heritable CJD, namely, after death, or postmortem, by brain autopsy.[41] Thus, no one directly or indirectly included in this narrative—not the physician, the mother, the rabbi or the daughter—could possibly have known the patient had heritable CJD within the timeframe of the tale, as told in the daughter's own words.

The pitfalls, and prejudices, of folk taxonomy

Following the tale's apparently fictitious rabbi, Liebman Jacobs recognized the narrator as a 'descendant' based on her mother's 'Sephardi' disease. What she did not recognize was the *FOAFtale* format, the tale's problematic timeframe, the fact that Libyan Jews cannot be swept into an over-inclusive Sephardi category or the fact that heritable CJD cannot be diagnosed before death, and has never been diagnosed among Spanish Americans or among descendants of Spanish Jews. Hence, it is important to stress, again, that when academics step out of their own areas of specialty they cease to be experts and revert to being ordinary folks, enabled and disabled by the same strengths and weaknesses of the universal human condition. In the case we have just seen, the academic author had no apparent training in the academic field she entered, a departure from her own area of specialty, which led her to discover crypto-Jewish 'descendants' wherever she sought them, and to slap 'Jewish' labels on ambiguous cultural paradigms across an entirely non-Jewish landscape.

It is therefore significant that scientists charged with identifying patterns within the human genome are themselves not trained to recognize the negative scientific and social consequences of labelling diseases according to non-heritable, essentially untestable cultural characteristics or according to demonstrably unfounded constructions of disease-based religious descent, as seen in the examples above. Moreover, from a scientific point of view, such folk taxonomies can seriously compromise fact-gathering, as well as

40 Ibid. (emphasis added).
41 Larry J. Lutwick, 'Creutzfeldt-Jakob disease', in Jacqueline L. Longe (ed.), *The Gale Encyclopedia of Medicine*, 2nd edn, 5 vols (Detroit: Gale Group 2002), ii.950–4 (953).

healthcare delivery, since they inevitably result in wishful, impressionistic—or academically misled—self-definition (as 'Jewish') by whole populations selected for genetic screening (or simply seeking it), based on non-heritable (as well as non-Jewish) traits and characteristics.

Yet, in the regional social context, it is clear that New Mexican folk-use of the term 'Jewish' for various and sundry heritable diseases serves only to strengthen a regional colour-coded hierarchy, maintained in perpetuity by ongoing claims of descent that both reflect and reinforce a pseudo-scientific social pathology, in this case, prejudicial, colonial tenets aided and abetted by seemingly 'innocent' academic authority. But the genetic labelling of faith communities can never be innocent, for faith communities are socially, not genetically, constructed and there is no such thing as a culturally constructed, 'congenital' line of religious affiliation that has no consequence in social stratification (for which modern New Mexico may be the best example).

As Mary Louise Pratt observes, it was colonial dominion, not genetic mapping, that first 'exerted the power' to name, or label, newly discovered populations:

> Indeed it was in naming that the religious and geographical projects came together, as emissaries claimed the world by baptizing landmarks and geographical formations with Euro-Christian names. But again, *natural history's naming is more directly transformative. It extracts all the things of the world and redeploys them into a new knowledge* ...[42]

We can see how giving names to categories in the natural world is itself a powerful form of classification, one that brings into being a hegemonic world order: a typically overarching, self-authenticating notion of 'the way things are'. Hence, to name biological groups according to religious affiliation is effectively to follow Linnaeus, not only by drawing genetic boundaries around cultural characteristics but also by transforming mutable religious affiliations into fixed congenital conditions. In this manner, all 'despised' or demonized characteristics assigned to religious Others are cast as biologically immutable, a highly precarious position for any vulnerable minority. In particular, given the over-generalized status of the category 'Jew', and knowing that over-inclusive folk logic is required to generate and sustain prejudice, it seems almost inevitable that academic classifications of heritable diseases as 'Jewish' will fan the flames of popular antisemitism. Moreover, if the label 'Jewish' is to be the only religious term associated with heritable disease, it can only bolster over-inclusive folk constructions of a singularly contaminated, and therefore a singularly contaminating, faith community. Gordon Allport never suggested that all over-inclusive cate-

42 Pratt, *Imperial Eyes*, 33 (emphasis added).

gories are necessarily prejudiced, only that they are undifferentiated and therefore pave the way for prejudice. To avoid paving that way, it may be helpful to distinguish between a mere misconception, and a *bona fide* prejudice. As he explains:

> Not every overblown generalization is a prejudice. Some are merely *misconceptions*, wherein we organize wrong information. ... Here we have the test to help us distinguish between ordinary errors of prejudgment and prejudice. If a person is capable of rectifying his erroneous judgments in the light of new evidence he is not prejudiced. *Prejudgments become prejudices only if they are not reversible when exposed to new knowledge*. A prejudice, unlike a simple misconception, is actively resistant to all evidence that would unseat it. We tend to grow emotional when a prejudice is threatened with contradiction. Thus the difference between ordinary prejudgments and prejudice is that one can discuss and rectify a prejudgment without emotional resistance.[43]

Like Linnaeus in an earlier age of discovery, we are suddenly called upon to define new categories of human variation and, when we are mistaken, to correct our misconceptions without prejudice. Unlike Linnaeus, we have greater hindsight and voluminous academic enlightenment to guide us. But, as we have seen, in our haste to name heritable disorders according to non-heritable characteristics, we are ourselves at risk of creating inaccurate, over-inclusive folk categories, foregoing academic accuracy and reinforcing our own self-authenticating social devices and/or those of historically preju-diced populations. As previously suggested, use of geographically based variance seems a more valid, reliable and socially responsible way of categorizing heritable differences, since every heritable disease has a founder who can be located in time and place: a testable assumption in every case, which cannot be said for any founder's religious sensibility. As Joseph Graves puts it: 'The practice of building whole theoretical constructs on essentially untestable assumptions is the hallmark of pseudo-science ... often associated with vested social agendas.'[44] Assuming that one's social agenda is benevolent and entirely well-meaning, there is still no agenda more benevolent than accuracy in distinguishing human populations or in practising health-related science. Therefore, to paraphrase Linneaus, the Ariadne thread in human classification is disciplined, differentiating academic logic, without which only chaos can prevail.

43 Allport, *The Nature of Prejudice*, 9.
44 Joseph L. Graves, Jr., *The Emperor's New Clothes: Biological Theories of Race at the Millennium* (New Brunswick, NJ: Rutgers University Press 2001), 87.

Judith S. Neulander is a folklorist. She is co-director of the Judaic Studies Program and teaches in the Department of Religious Studies at Case Western Reserve University in Cleveland, Ohio. Her award-winning doctoral research discredited claims of a crypto-Jewish survival in New Mexico, but her primary research *foci* include science and religion, folklore and religion, and traditional arts and architectures. She has published widely on these topics, has earned an Emmy nomination as an associate producer of folklore segments for PBS, and has created a number of museum exhibitions across the country. She is frequently invited to publish on the subject of *ersatz* crypto-Jews and has written the entry on the subject in the new edition of the *Encyclopedia of American Folklife* (M. E. Sharpe 2006). She lectures in the United States and abroad, and is currently working on three books.

Eugenics and the racial genome: politics at the molecular level

SHARON L. SNYDER AND DAVID T. MITCHELL

ABSTRACT   Snyder and Mitchell's essay charts parallels between the historical marginalization of disabled populations and that of racialized populations, including the overlap in experiences of disability. It then assesses ways in which the history of the US eugenics movement can serve as a predictor of outcomes for projects like the Genomic Research of the African Diaspora biobank (GRAD) at Howard University, which attempt to trace genetic markers for disability prevalent in African-American communities. Diagnostic practices at the population level have previously threatened to entrench forms of pathology at the biological level without delivering promised relief through the discovery of cures. Specifically, the eugenics movement undertook restrictive measures to manage those deemed 'genetically inferior'. While it promised that widespread diagnostic labels would lead to the end of severe disabilities—particularly mental 'subnormality'—the movement failed to lessen levels of disability at the same time as it deflected needed social support away from disabled people. As a result, disabled peoples' historical devaluation resulted in the loss of key citizenship privileges, such as freedom to move about the country, reproductive participation and the right to live in the community. While diagnostic initiatives might begin with a seemingly benign intention to alleviate disability as 'suffering', medical labels often result in a further level of social disenfranchisement for members of the target population. Despite historical differences between genetics and eugenics, Snyder and Mitchell argue that similar outcomes are likely to result from racialized genomic research undertaken in minority communities in the United States.

The limits of biology

The fact that disabled people share histories of discrimination, marginalization and civil rights-based struggles with other racial minority groups in the United States is little discussed. These histories are intertwined—often to a substantial degree—but run on parallel tracks because the integrity of one's own marginalization can seem diminished when it intersects with that of another. This essay probes the relationship between eugenics-based applications as they cross-reference disability and racial 'inferiority'. If the historian of racism George Fredrickson proves to be correct, racism can be historicized as a relatively recent, and thus historically finite, phenomenon.[1] Likewise, disability disenfranchisement also appears no more than 200 or 300 years old.[2] Consequently, we want to suggest that these two forms of 'body-based' disqualification—according to which a population's access to influential cultural privileges and institutions is understood to be 'innate' and therefore inevitable—share a surprisingly intimate lineage in western discursive traditions.[3] Not in the sense of having been subject to interchangeable kinds of mistreatment and segregation strategies, but rather that both groups' exploitation having been the result of an attendant incapacity. The notion of this deficiency, termed 'in-built inferiority' by Fredrickson, is based on the idea that a group's shortcomings are biologically encoded and cannot be transcended to any significant degree.[4]

Recently, some of the coordinates of this shared experience between African Americans and people with disabilities came to light during a day-long summit held in Salt Lake City, Utah on the dual status of disability and race. According to the *Salt Lake City Tribune*, the summit revealed that 'both groups say they face similar hurdles such as poverty, discrimination, lack of political clout and, sometimes, a public backlash created by perceptions that they get special treatment. Many also share a fear that they cannot find help or afford services.'[5] Importantly, the summit helped to identify a series of little discussed 'hurdles' that both groups face despite divergent historical origins of discrimination. While a transatlantic slave trade forms the foundation of African-American discrimination, for instance, disabled people's devaluation results largely from a history of institutionalization and reproductive control. However, divergent causes do not preclude an investigation into the shared social rationale that reinforces explanations of why neither population 'thrives' in a social sense. There may be some

1 George M. Fredrickson, *Racism: A Short History* (Princeton, NJ: Princeton University Press 2002).
2 Deborah A. Stone, *The Disabled State* (Philadelphia: Temple University Press 1984).
3 We pursue a parallel argument about the intimate relationship between body-based discrimination towards racial populations and that towards disability populations in our recent book *Cultural Locations of Disability* (Chicago and London: University of Chicago Press 2006). In particular, see chapter three, 'The Eugenic Atlantic', for a discussion of the advent of pathologies that cannot be transcended by any degree of cultural training. The argument here is not intended to juxtapose racial and disability systems of exclusion as being one and the same, but rather to compare the influence of eugenics discourse on the cultural rationale that devalues both groups in a similar manner.
4 Fredrickson, *Racism*, 3.
5 B. Griggs, 'Dual status of disability, race studies', *Salt Lake City Tribune*, 3 October 2003, B2.

significant lessons to be drawn from the paralleling of these two groups, particularly in that disability (unlike gender or race) can be experienced by any societal grouping at any time.

Speaking to this precise point, the author of the *Salt Lake City Tribune* article ends with a hope that the next summit will attract racial minorities *with* disabilities. Race and disability continue to be imagined as mutually distinct phenomena rather than as overlapping moments of social oppression, particularly given that the long history of biological racism grounding arguments about African-American inferiority also influences characterizations of disabled people.[6] A eugenics-informed logic about intellectual inferiority has served as the guiding rationale for both groups' inability to function in a competitive market-based economy. The voicelessness of both groups on issues pertaining to their own social welfare might be added as yet another shared characteristic of their contemporary social situations.

Both groups, in effect, share a social atmosphere that presumes limits of biology (especially limited intelligence) as the source of a population's disqualification. While statistics on the situation of racial minority groups are now generally well known, those detailing the situation of people with disabilities *of all races* may be less familiar. Currently, disabled people's social demographics include the following: 69 per cent of disabled people were unemployed in 2002 (the highest figure in twenty years); 1.9 million disabled people are currently housed in institutions; employers win nearly 96 per cent of all disability-based discrimination lawsuits filed under the Americans with Disabilities Act; the national average rent for a one-bedroom apartment now exceeds the average monthly income of people with disabilities; disabled people are victims of crime at rates 4–10 times higher than for non-disabled people; disabled people's treatment is unduly characterized by objectification by the rehabilitation and medical industries; and, finally, people with disabilities face rampant discrimination in public housing due to a paucity of accessible, affordable living spaces.[7] These statistics provide an overview of a population demographic that is actually composed of individuals that have little in common with each other medically or physiologically. However, the statistics point to shared social experiences based on stigmatizing attitudes towards bodily/ cognitive differences and the threatened eclipse of one's humanity by medical labels.

Not only will one find a constellation of negative social experiences that is shared between racial and disabled groups. But Howard University's Genomic Research of the African Diaspora (GRAD) project and a host of other biobanks promise to deepen the historical relationship between race and

6 Snyder and Mitchell, *Cultural Locations of Disability.*
7 National Council on Disability (NCD), *National Disability Policy: A Progress Report December 2000–December 2001* (Washington, D.C.: NCD 2002).

disability at the molecular level.[8] As we read into the reporting of this new initiative (and our observations here are going to be based primarily on the journalistic translation of these 'scientific' issues), we find that GRAD intends to eliminate the health disparity between African Americans and other demographic groups, particularly those of European (white) derivation. By creating a database of African-American genetic composition, researchers of GRAD hope to identify disease rates, disability prevalence and health indexes that characterize 'black experience' in the United States. Since 'health' professionals and researchers believe significant disparities exist between African Americans and other demographic groups, GRAD seeks to close the gap in medical knowledge by specifically targeting the health of African Americans by means of a racially specific genetic-sampling effort.

However, one quickly discovers that the resulting genetic database will not be a 'racial' sampling of African Americans. Rather, cheek swabs will be taken from a specific racialized population, namely, the patients found in Howard University's affiliated hospitals and area clinics.[9] And neither will the genetic sampling be based on the general hospital population, but on a more specific group, primarily African Americans with disabilities. The trinity of disorders most commonly cited in the literature as potentially benefitting from the databank include hypertension, diabetes and prostate cancer, and sometimes obesity and renal failure are mentioned as well.[10] These conditions are believed to affect African Americans disproportion-ately, just as Tay Sachs syndrome has a purported prevalence among certain Jewish populations. Thus, we are now on the cusp of a new era of identifying racial groups on the basis of shared markers for certain genetic mutations considered deleterious by medical researchers.

Much of the journalistic coverage of GRAD to date has cited widespread mistrust among African-American communities of clinical research and medical researchers as a key obstacle to the gathering of reliable data.[11] The suspicion that health professionals are not working in their best interests is also found in disability communities, which often believe medicine and clinical research settings to be the ground zero of their social stigma. Among African Americans the most commonly cited source of this distrust is the Tuskeegee Institute experiments,[12] in which 399 black men with syphilis went

8 Avram Goldstein and Rick Weiss, 'Howard U. plans genetics database: school says data on African Americans could lead to better medical care', *Washington Post*, 28 May 2003, A06; Jocelyn Kaiser, 'African-American population biobank proposed', *Science*, vol. 300, 6 June 2003, 1485.

9 Andrew Pollack, 'DNA of Blacks to be gathered to fight illness', *New York Times*, 27 May 2003, A1; Goldstein and Weiss, 'Howard U. plans genetic database'; Kaiser, 'African-American population biobank proposed'.

10 Goldstein and Weiss, 'Howard U. plans genetic database'.

11 Pollack, 'DNA of Blacks to be gathered to fight illness'; Goldstein and Weiss, 'Howard U. plans genetic database'.

12 Kaiser, 'African-American population biobank proposed'.

deliberately untreated for four decades, from 1932 to 1972, and more than 100 died directly or indirectly as a result.[13] However, we want to argue that the Tuskeegee example is more pertinent to a history of abuses in medical experimentation. This is terrain shared with people with disabilities who have been subject to such institutional experiments, including children with mental retardation being fed cereal in which radioactive milk has been added (we'll return to this parallel later). With respect to GRAD's racial biobank project, however, the last time such an effort was made to gather condition-based information on a mass scale on behalf of science was at the time of the eugenics movement. It is to that movement that we may most effectively look for precedents on a similar scale to current human genome projects as well as the potential outcomes of an international diagnostic campaign.

Our contention is that health-based comparisons based on tracking disability rates result in the targeted populations in question being stigmatized. First, disability is not the antithesis of 'health', as these studies assume. Instead, genetically based differences result in bodies/minds that deviate from a naturalized norm of capacity, function and/or appearance. When one tracks disability rates one does not chart occurrences of 'ill health', but rather varying manifestations of biological variation. A disabled body, within this argument, is not the flip side of a 'healthy' body; rather, it represents part of the range of variation that regularly surfaces across a dynamic species. Disabled bodies are those bodies (as is the case with all bodies) in the process of establishing their own norms of functionality and typicality. These norms may diverge significantly from members of a 'generically' identified population, but one does not measure deviance in 'health status' when one follows disability rates.

Sciences of the universal and the local

Human genome based research has pursued two distinct trajectories: first, the 'mapping' of the full sequence of the human genome in order to identify a universal paradigm of genetic data; and, second, including projects such as GRAD, a more 'essentialist' effort to identify the specific genetic make-up of particular migratory groups. In the case of the former, the effort is primarily 'empirical' in that it is driven by a largely ahistorical attempt to discover what Ian Hacking has called an 'indifferent kind', that is, a universal type shorn of environmental influence.[14] The second project, the 'universalist paradigm', is best exemplified by the 'gold standard' argument in genomics in which chromosomal anomalies are intentionally dropped out of DNA

13 See Susan M. Reverby (ed.), *Tuskeegee's Truths: Rethinking the Tuskeegee Syphilis Study* (Chapel Hill: University of North Carolina Press 2000).
14 Ian Hacking, *The Social Construction of What?* (Cambridge, MA: Harvard University Press 2000).

sequencing patterns in order to identify an 'unsullied' genetic core that no single individual possesses. In this case, what we will refer to here as the 'diversity approach', the effort becomes one of generational filiation in which a people's ancestry can be traced back through their chromosomal heritage. A striking example of this methodology, otherwise referred to as tracing genetic drift, was reported in an *Atlantic Monthly* article in 2001.[15] Geneticists at Stanford University traced the migration of a genetically 'mutated' Y chromosome, which 'appears in more than half of all Native American males', back across the Bering Straits to its origin in Korea.

While these two seemingly opposing approaches may appear antithetical, they evolve out of a shared impetus: the identification of genetic 'deviance' tells us simultaneously what is most 'typical' and what is most distinctive about human populations. In this sense, both disabled people during the heyday of the eugenics movement and black Americans with genetic conditions now are sources of information about their bodies that medical knowledge can use to benefit the 'rest of us'.

During the main eugenics period (which we will date here as running from the 1880s to the 1930s in the United States), a massive research campaign was carried out on the bodies and lifestyles of people labelled 'feebleminded'. In order to be clear, a designation of 'feeblemindedness' was not limited to individuals with cognitive disabilities. It also included individuals with sensory impairments such as deafness and blindness, those with a variety of congenital physical impairments (such as epilepsy, cerebral palsy and muscular dystrophy), immigrants trying to master English as their non-native tongue, racialized peoples, as well as those identified as criminals, delinquents, schizophrenics and the sexually ambiguous. Perhaps most importantly, 'feeblemindedness' designated bodies that presented combinations of these characteristics. With respect to immigrant classes, Isabelle Thompson Smart, a New York physician-inspector, wrote in 1912:

> In every instance I found positive physical defects, and, with many, a combination of physical unfitness with a serious mental defect, which demanded a proper segregation of the case in question ... The greater number of the physical defects could be very much bettered—many of them cured—but the mental unfitness is irreparable. Up to a certain point, all of these cases could be trained to become useful units in a colony life, suited to their individual needs and under proper supervision; but if left to drift, after their brief term of school life ends, will in large measure become derelicts, and will, in time, fill our penal institutions and our homes for fallen women or worse, live at large and procreate their kind in large numbers.[16]

15 Steve Olson, 'The genetic archaeology of race', *Atlantic Monthly*, April 2001, 69–80.
16 Isabelle Thompson Smart, 'Studies in relation of physical inability and mental deficiency to the body social', in *Transactions of the Fifteenth International Congress in Hygiene and Demography. Washington, DC, 23–8 September, 1912* (Washington, D.C.: GPO 1913), 1–8.

Ironically, because African Americans were presumed to be of inferior intelligence as a result of their race, they largely escaped the devastating impact of institutionalized eugenics until the late 1940s.[17] Some race scholars have argued that this 'exemption' from widespread institutionalization provides further proof of racism—particularly in the American South—and this is an accurate contention. There was a racist ideology at work in the belief that African-American populations were so intellectually inferior that institutionalization would be unrealistic. One eugenic study of 'feeblemind-edness' in the South reported in 1919 that upwards of 93 per cent of all black children in one Georgia county had tested as 'intellectually subnormal'.[18] However, one is left wondering if the racial discrimination that prevented thousands of African Americans from being institutionalized (as was the case for their disabled counterparts among Caucasian and other non-black populations) proved to be more of a blessing in disguise. Gaining better access to the country's institutional structures—particularly those devoted to the determination of a root cause for defining human differences—can have its drawbacks.

From external defects to internal flaws

Of course, to compare any contemporary research initiative to eugenics practices of the past is to invite the charge of historical slander. In order to avoid this unflattering historical association between eugenics and genetics, the Human Genome Project (HGP) has adopted two anticipatory tactics with respect to the media. On the one hand, the HGP has cannily positioned its coverage in the media in relation to the promise of genetic cures, the moral foundation of the research. On the other hand, the HGP has employed aggressive opinion polls that query a public about its anti-science leanings as a means of pre-empting an anticipated backlash against genetic data-gathering. In this article, we do not wish simply to equate eugenics with the HGP or its various spin-offs, such as GRAD, but rather to draw some parallels and distinctions that need to be made at the outset. Particularly given that our chosen disability studies methodology seeks to demonstrate what social and cultural models of disability might contribute to this discussion.

The previous century's eugenic science resulted in the active disenfranch-isement of disabled people (and those labelled 'disabled') from levels of participation and experience afforded to most other citizens. Eugenics was

17 Steven Noll, *Feeble-minded in Our Midst: Institutions for the Mentally Retarded in the South, 1900–1940* (Chapel Hill: University of North Carolina Press 1995).
18 V. V. Anderson, 'Mental defect in a southern state: report of the Georgia Commission on Feeblemindedness and the survey of the National Committee on Mental Hygiene', *Mental Hygiene*, vol. 3, no. 4, October 1919, 527–65.

not a link in the chain of complicity to designate disabled people as 'defective', but rather the fence itself, which limited the freedoms and mobility of its target population. Thus, one of the most celebrated modernist novels, William Faulkner's *The Sound and the Fury*, begins with a thirty-three-year-old man with Down Syndrome named Benjy walking within a fenced enclosure. Benjy is accompanied by his African-American caretaker charged with keeping him from bothering the golfers on the other side of the fence. Eugenicists participated in a quintessentially modernist project, whose *modus operandi* consisted of efforts to classify and pathologize human differences now referred to as 'disabilities'. While often parading under the humanist guise of assistance to 'the unfortunate', 'the suffering' and 'the unfit', eugenics accomplished its debilitating effects through the deployment of taxonomies of naming, the statistical calculation of average and non-standard bodies and, particularly, through participation in normative science. The eugenics period provided the tools and rationale that fuelled a hygienic drive towards the valorization of a largely unquestioned biological standardization.

In brief, disability studies remains entirely aware that eugenics was not an aberration of modernism, as the majority of the 'ethical' projects funded by the HGP claim: merely the effort to implement a 'bad idea', as one HGP-funded study explains. By putting aside a much celebrated 5 per cent of all research funds to examine ethical issues, the HGP has effectively navigated a canny name change from 'eugenics' to 'genetics' since the 1950s. While the shift in nomenclature appears relatively minor, genetics has succeeded in placing an enormous amount of distance between its objectives and those of its predecessor science. Genetics has effectively accomplished what intellectual historian John Limon describes as science's penchant for cannibalizing its own past.[19] In doing so, eugenics approaches to prevention, population management, sorting and adjudicating bodily hierarchies remain an unacknowledged part of our own era's scientific methodology. Along with an expanded understanding of genetics and an adept public rhetoric, genome research has managed to retain many of the methods of its predecessor.

In particular, this can be seen with respect to genetic science's approach to disabling conditions, in that the underlying mechanisms of bodies continue to be identified as the appropriate site of 'intervention'. Yet, no money from genetics has gone towards support for people living with disabilities in hostile social environments created for bodies with certain capacities. This emphasis is most evident in the fervent predictions about genetic cures. A gene location is 'discovered' and its identification quickly leads to predictions of 'effective interventions'. Yet, in nearly every case, these predications quickly transform into practices of 'prevention' (i.e. forms of

19 John Limon, *The Place of Fiction in the Time of Science* (Cambridge: Cambridge University Press 1990).

screening that provide opportunities to abort foetuses with maligned markers). For instance, disability studies scholars such as Tim Stainton have argued that genetic testing essentially bestows a disability-based identity on an unborn foetus in that parents contemplate whether to abort based on their knowledge (or lack of knowledge) of living people with that diagnostic label.[20] Adrienne Asch argues that parental decisions are based on too little information about disability and therefore a positive genetic screen for Down Syndrome (for instance) often calls up social stigmas and stereotypes foreign to friends and families of people living with the condition in question.[21] How can genetic counselling encourage individual choice in these cases when the decisions are so often based on stigmatized public attitudes towards disabled individuals or, in the case of foetuses with positive disability screenings, proto-individuals?

In order to gather data for its scientific efforts to trace the hereditary impact of 'defective' gene stocks, eugenics employed a number of tools and methods aimed at identifying those who possessed inferior 'genes' (or 'germ plasm' as the nomenclature of the day had it). First and foremost was a conception of aggregate population traits developed out of the discipline of statistics. Accordingly, large pools of quantitative sampling data were translated into the well-known bell curve scenario. The most reproduced traits were represented in the bulky middle of the curve and the more rare or anomalous traits spread out to comprise right and left tails. Eugenics sought to influence the distribution of traits across a population artificially by selecting out and sex-segregating or sterilizing those thought to possess 'defective genes'. The HGP, minus an open collusion with state-sponsored segregation and sterilization policies, continues this effort to use science in order to engineer an alternative distribution of hereditary traits across populations.

As in the case of formal racism, the lack of coordinated collaboration between science and severely restrictive public policies has begun to place some distance between today's genetics and yesterday's eugenics. Yet, as we pointed out in our opening statistics, institutionalization still remains a significant threat to the freedom of 1.9 million disabled people. Less publicly available is the persistence of sterilization options utilized on disabled people. Significant evidence exists to suggest that disabled people are coerced into sterilization operations as a form of 'therapy' or in exchange for their freedom from institutions. There is also a common story that surfaces among disabled women in which they undergo surgery in their adolescent

---

20 Tim Stainton, 'Identity, difference and the ethical politics of prenatal testing', *Journal of Intellectual Disability Research*, vol. 47, no. 7, October 2003, 533–9.

21 Adrienne Asch, 'Why I haven't changed my mind about prenatal diagnosis: reflections and refinements', in Erik Parens and Adrienne Asch (eds), *Prenatal Testing and Disability Rights* (Washington, D.C.: Georgetown University Press 2000), 234–58.

years for one procedure only to learn that they have received hysterectomies. Whereas eugenics systematically endorsed sterilization as 'treatment', we are now in an era of more clandestine practices that prove difficult to trace. Many eugenic attitudes remain intact but the lessening of state enforcement helps to shape a new historical apparatus. Moreover, our lack of open discussion about the impact of eugenics in the United States (as opposed to a country such as Germany) ensures that little understanding exists with respect to the proximity of today's genetics to discriminatory beliefs of the late nineteenth and early twentieth centuries.

The most extreme interventionist project—the *failed* effort to identify and prevent the transmission of undesirable traits—was largely championed by eugenicists who believed that even the median (i.e. most replicated) characteristics of a population tended to express evolutionary regression overall. It is important to keep this point in mind because today's genetics must ultimately be assessed on the basis of its attitude towards *the overall genetic composition of its populations*. As soon as one witnesses a rhetorical shift towards generalized regression in the genetic make-up of a country, one may effectively assume that we are in the domain of eugenics.

However, if one's genomic research bank is based, from the beginning, on a sampling of disabled people of colour, isn't genome research reading backwards? In other words, doesn't our contemporary willingness to designate inherently undesirable traits on the surface already presume that we will ultimately discover a regressive genetic system on the inside? This question is presumably left open for genetic research to answer, but one would be hard pressed to imagine that this will not prove the case. In any case, this is exactly the direction in which the diagnostic gaze of eugenics moved: from undesirable exterior to inferior interior.

Human hereditary pedigrees

Like GRAD and other human genome based research projects, eugenics went far beyond the designation of disability and disease at an individual level. Elaborate *human pedigree charts* were constructed in order to trace the passage of 'defective' traits genealogically from one generation to another. Michel Foucault refers to this as the slandering of entire genetic genera-tions.[22] Because this project was based on a relatively simplistic model of dominant-recessive Mendelian genetics, eugenicists believed that an aber-rant trait in one generation (such as epilepsy) could be transformed into an alternative expression of defect in a later generation (such as 'feebleminded-ness'). Consequently, one could use a pedigree chart to map the linear

22 Michel Foucault, *Abnormal: Lectures at the Collège de France, 1974–1975*, ed. Valerio Marchetti and Antonella Salomoni, trans. from the French by Graham Burchell (New York: Picador 2003), 313.

generational transfer of defective traits that actually bore little genetic relationship to one another. In addition, much of the 'data' contained in eugenics pedigree charts was based on hearsay. For instance, a neighbour might remark to an interviewer on the 'strangeness' or 'slowness' of a now dead relative, and that comment would be enough to allow a probability of 'feeblemindedness' to be recorded as the determining characteristic of the extinct individual in question. The HGP initiative may be involved in more informed assumptions about the genetic basis of disorders, but it still produces the equivalent of human pedigree charts when it maps genetic data for individuals, generations or populations.

Eugenics set a precedent for what can happen when a massive scientific and public health campaign is conducted on an international scale. Not only were people with disabilities synonymous with groups found to be universally deficient in some shared characteristic, but many countries began exchanging statistics on percentages of defective individuals living within their borders. In fact, so much deleterious research about disability was exported back and forth across the Atlantic between the United States, Britain, France, Germany, the Netherlands and various colonial outposts that we have called the site of this collaborative effort the 'Eugenic Atlantic', an allusion to Paul Gilroy's 1993 work on the trafficking of race, *The Black Atlantic*.[23] Just as beliefs in racial inferiority bolstered economic and ideological commerce between Europe and the Americas from the sixteenth to the nineteenth centuries, shared notions of disability have enhanced investments in acceptable bodies from the late nineteenth century onwards.

The development of tens of thousands of human pedigree charts on inmates housed in institutions for the 'feebleminded' during the eugenics period also demonstrates the mass nature of this 'mapping' campaign. Some of the first female scientists were employed by eugenics researchers to put a 'soft face' on this masculinist science. Because eugenics targeted 'feeble-minded' women in particular, the belief was that women fieldworkers would tend to allay the suspicions of the family and friends of the 'diagnosed'. White, middle-class female fieldworkers were recruited to provide the venture with a 'maternal' interest in the well-being of families identified as objects of eugenic intervention (largely lower-class, Caucasian and other non-black families with at least one institutionalized family member).

One may witness both of these aspects potentially at work in the GRAD project. For instance, in order to lessen suspicion of clinical trials in black communities, the Howard University project is based on research conducted by African-American professionals and researchers. This is not to dispute

23   David T. Mitchell and Sharon L. Snyder, 'Eugenic Atlantic: race, disability, and the making of an international eugenic science, 1800–1945', *Disability & Society*, vol. 18, no. 7, December 2003, 843–64; Paul Gilroy, *The Black Atlantic: Modernity and Double Consciousness* (Cambridge, MA: Harvard University Press 2005).

the fact that African-American institutions should have access to mega-million-dollar research projects like the HGP. Rather, it is to argue that involving predominantly African-American institutions in this effort does not guarantee the beneficence of the ultimate research findings. If race is constructed, can we expect a middle-class professional coterie of African Americans necessarily to put the best interests of its subjects first, as is claimed in numerous articles? The Tuskeegee experiments demonstrate that Eunice Rivers, Eugene Dibble and other African-American professionals could not resist becoming complicit in the medical deception in which disability and/or class mitigated against racial solidarity. Essentialist premises of this kind may benefit a black professional class, but that benefit does not automatically trickle down to the subjects of the research, particularly the largely impoverished black citizens with disabilities whose DNA is to be included in the biobank.

Many scholars suspicious of the HGP have warned that the discounting of the diverse biological and social influences impacting genetics threatens to underwrite a new myth of biology-is-destiny in discourses of the genome. Rather than defining genes as a site of replication and bookkeeping, genetics diminishes the role of the environment in favour of genes being defined as causal agents in species development. This critique of genetics' over-emphasis on the building blocks of life is taken up by the late Stephen Jay Gould in his work *The Structure of Evolutionary Theory*. For Gould there was little question that 'genes influence organisms; one might even say, metaphorically to be sure, that genes act as blueprints to build organisms', but this does not mean that they are causal agents in their own right:

> [Genetics] commits one of the classical errors in historical reasoning by arguing that because genes preceded organisms in time, and then aggregated to form cells and organisms, genes must therefore control organisms—[this is] a confusion of historical priority with current domination.[24]

This genetic obfuscation of the levels of agency is crucial in that it encourages public misrecognition of appropriate sites for intervention. Population genomics seeks data in order to continue identifying sequence strands that manifest undesirable traits. Any eventual focus will involve changing bodies, particularly in cases of mutation that are often defined by their random, sudden and inevitable appearances.

In contradistinction to the emphasis on bodily interventions in genetics, disability constituencies ask that we work to change inaccessible environments and social structures, rather than a still largely unavailable biological core. This shift in focus would show our commitment to current generations of individuals living with disabilities who are excluded from full participa-

24 Stephen Jay Gould, *The Structure of Evolutionary Theory* (Cambridge, MA: Belknap Press of Harvard University Press 2002), 618.

tion by social obstacles and attitudinal barriers. Environments and attitudes are infinitely more malleable than human organisms; yet, the
genetics gambit is based on an inversion of this principle. Most of all,
genetics threatens to participate in the reduction of human cultures and
experiences to diagnostic labels, insisting more fervently than most movements in medical history that a disorder mandate one's oversight in a
medical destiny.

Genetic knowledge will not allow a stripping away of difference. In fact, it
will provoke a confrontation with a series of serious ethical and moral
questions, particularly those that have been noted by scholars in disabilities
studies for at least the past decade. For instance, one of the staple arguments
of the disability rights movement has been that aborting a foetus based on
disability status deepens the stigma against those living with the same
conditions.[25] Many scholars have pointed out that the hyperbolic rhetoric of
'cure' that abounds in genetics and in the journalistic coverage of the
field has grave social repercussions for the status of contemporary disabled
people. As more funds pour into curative sciences, less is provided for
supporting those with disabilities. Human pedigree mapping underwrites a
purely diagnostic impetus that has yet to deliver on the curative premises of
its presumed intervention. In the meantime, just as at the time of the
eugenics movement, more and more bodies are found wanting in their
make-up as society continues to emphasize identification over meaningful
integration.

Why do disability communities want a voice at the genome table?

Research conducted on behalf of disabled persons or on behalf of a social
order that is burdened with their existence cannot effectively value human
differences considered a priori 'unliveable' or 'tragic'. Without the centrality
of the perspectives of people living with disabilities, we are bound to
reproduce narratives about their conditions that are both inaccurate and
socially debilitating. Further, if we understand that racism and ablism
continue to persist, how can projects such as GRAD avoid the discriminatory
referencing across racial and disability lines that bolster social perceptions of
inferiority?

The hyperbolic rhetoric about disability experiences that permeate the
conduct of research and funding create visions of grotesque suffering for
dramatic effect. In order to generate funding stocks to undertake such efforts
there has been an unnecessary ratcheting up of rhetoric about conditions 'too
horrible to imagine'. For instance, one of the authors' disability has been

25 International League of Societies for Persons with Mental Handicap (ILSMH), *The
Beliefs, Values and Principles of Self-Advocacy* (Brussels: ILSMH 1994); Parens and Asch
(eds), *Prenatal Testing and Disability Rights*.

recently described as 'horribly crippling' by the *Chicago Tribune*.[26] There appears to be some mutation in the language of genetics that encourages such monstrous flourishes of discourse.

'Cure talk' has become 'prevention talk'. Population-wide promises make the persistence of disabilities seem a matter of individual culpability rather than a failure of modern science to live up to its up prophecies. Eugenics made similar promises and attached a belief in modern advancement to their fulfillment.

A half-century's worth of genetic promises had an effect on generations of children with disabilities who went ahead and grew up without waiting for genetics to 'complete' them. However, in their wake, disabled people have carried on through degrees of stigma and public inaccessibility that have prevented their meaningful participation. The voices of disabled people need to be heard not only in consultations about genetics but also in the production of the knowledge base. We need a genetics industry that will openly pursue the professionalization of disabled people in the name of the science that disproportionately impacts their lives. Finally and at the very least, disabled people need an honest acknowledgement by the genetics leaders that, without their genetic uniqueness, our understanding of genes and genetics would be much less advanced.

Sharon L. Snyder and **David T. Mitchell** are both members of the faculty of the Ph.D. programme in disability studies and the Department of Disability and Human Development at the University of Illinois at Chicago. They have co-authored four books on the history, art and culture of people with disabilities, including *The Body and Physical Difference* (1997), *Narrative Prosthesis* (2000), *The Encyclopedia of Disability* (5 volumes, 2005) and *Cultural Locations of Disability* (2006). They have also produced four award-winning films: *Vital Signs: Crip Culture Talks Back* (1996), *A World without Bodies* (2002), *Self Preservation: The Art of Riva Lehrer* (2004) and *Disability Takes on the Arts* (2005). They are currently at work on a catalogue to accompany the Chicago Disability History exhibit.

26 Paul Elias, 'Gene map hasn't yet led to a big pay off', *Chicago Tribune*, 27 January 2003.

The risky gene: epidemiology and the evolution of race

PHILIP ALCABES

ABSTRACT   Alcabes examines how modern epidemiology views race, including a historical review and a critique of methods. Race occupies a central place in health discourse partly because of two misapprehensions. First, contemporary epidemiologic research focuses on individual behaviour as a determinant of disease risk, despite the fact that risk as predicted from epidemiologic data is solely interpretable for large populations, not for individuals. Historically and today, connections between behaviour and disease have been used to fortify racial discrimination, with reprobate behaviours imputed to unwanted races. Second, the advent of evolutionary theory and the recognition that genetics provides a mechanism by which evolution proceeds together have allowed for the social concept of 'race' to be imbued fallaciously with biological determinants. With an epidemiology based on behaviour, a behavioural indexing of race and a racial interpretation of evolutionary theory and genomics, the circle closes: society can ascribe differences in disease occurrence to the genetic make-up of the sufferers or to their behaviour, or both—that is, to race—and avoid having to address social problems that typically underlie disease risk.

The United States is the only industrialized nation that does not collect health data according to economic class.[1] Instead, we report almost every morbidity and mortality statistic by race. Yet, to elucidate how race figures in American epidemiology is a daunting task. We epidemiologists have yet to define what we mean when we examine 'race' (or 'ethnicity', as we usually call it now). And the epidemiologic literature is hot with controversy over how to handle race in health research.

While it would be an oversimplification to declare that there are only two positions in the debate about health and race, two core diametrically opposed positions are clear enough: one side holds that only if health researchers cease to keep track of race can the United States move past

---

1 Vicente Navarro, 'Race or class versus race and class: mortality differentials in the United States', in Dan E. Beauchamp and Bonnie Steinbock (eds), *New Ethics for the Public's Health* (New York and Oxford: Oxford University Press 1999), 39–44.

Black–White polarization.[2] The other contends that data *must* be arrayed by race because the field of public health must seek to understand how racism affects health.[3] Much is to be learned from each of the two main positions, and a few commentators have tried to make sense of them in ways that are enlightening. But I see no easy path to resolving the issue of race in health research.

Instead, I hope to show the central place that race occupies in American discourse and that discord has been shaped by two misapprehensions pertaining to disease. First, we have misread the epidemiologic concept of *risk*, thinking it applies to individual behaviour. Second, we have misread *evolution*, thinking it means that some genes are better than others. The concurrent emergence of both epidemiologic and evolutionary science, about 150 years ago, offered a seeming substantiation of race-thinking just when people in western societies were beginning to consider what to do about epidemic illness.

Risk

The epidemiologic meaning of risk is well defined: it is a probability claim, the odds that a member of a given population—Chicagoans, say—will come down with a given disease in the coming year. I can tell you that the risk of someone in that city dying of pneumonia or influenza in the coming year is on the order of 464 in a million. To epidemiologists, risk is a guess. That is why we usually hedge our bets, by stating risk as a *vicinity*: we use the so-called 95 per cent confidence interval, within which the probability of disease probably sits. I might say that the risk of dying of pneumonia or influenza in Chicago lies *somewhere between* 255 in a million and 826 in a million. I produced those probability estimates in the usual epidemiologist's way, the same way that a good player of horses figures out which horse to bet on: by looking at what happened in the past. In my case, I used data

2 The argument was articulated by Mindy Fullilove in 'Comment: abandoning "race" as a variable in public health research—an idea whose time has come', *American Journal of Public Health*, vol. 88, 1998, 1297–8. Others have offered rationales for related approaches, for instance, James Y. Nazroo, 'The structuring of ethnic inequalities in health: economic position, racial discrimination, and racism', *American Journal of Public Health*, vol. 93, 2003, 277–84.

3 Nancy Krieger sets forth the argument in 'Does racism harm health? Did child abuse exist before 1962? On explicit questions, critical science, and current controversies: an ecosocial perspective', *American Journal of Public Health*, vol. 93, 2003, 94–9. Camara Phyllis Jones offers a prescription for how to address racism in 'Invited commentary: "race," racism, and the practice of epidemiology', *American Journal of Epidemiology*, vol. 154, no. 4, 2001, 299–304. See also Nancy Krieger,' Discrimination and health', in Lisa F. Berkman and Ichiro Kawachi (eds), *Social Epidemiology* (New York and Oxford: Oxford University Press 2000), 36–75.

published by the United States Centers for Disease Control and Prevention (CDC), showing that there were 1,300 or so pneumonia-influenza deaths in Chicago in each of the last few years.[4] I calculated the vicinity estimate using probabilities figured out a couple of hundred years ago by the French mathematician Siméon Denis Poisson, based on *his* observations of past rare events.

Any good player of horses knows intuitively—and probably without ever having read David Hume on inference—that the past can never tell you the absolute truth about what is going to happen in the future. Sometimes you bet on the favourite and your horse loses to the longshot. This year's pneumonia-influenza death rate might be higher than I predicted, since nobody can predict exactly what is going to happen in nature. But, over time, what happened in the past is more likely than not to happen in the future as well. So, the player of horses is comfortable placing bets based on his scan of the past-performance charts, and the epidemiologist is comfortable making predictions about risk—stating probabilities, that is—when she has had a chance to observe diseases in large and stable populations over a longish period of time.

But we must also recognize what epidemiology cannot do. Our risk estimation process will not work well for small populations, and it does not work for an individual. Based on the data for the city of Chicago, I certainly would not try to predict how many of the baseball players sitting in the dugouts in Wrigley Field on a given day in July will die of pneumonia in the coming year. People are simply too different one from another to allow us to assume that one group's risk is the same as another's. This is intuitive, too: most of us would not assume that we can skateboard down staircases or over concrete barriers without injury to limb or loss of life just because we see our crazy children doing it.

Since epidemiologists do not always communicate well what we mean by risk, though, what we do transmit is misinterpreted much, maybe most, of the time. The biggest reason for this miscommunication is that epidemiology has turned its attention away from what it is best suited to, namely, studying how the forces of nature, the structure of society and the imperatives of economic systems affect the distribution of disease. This is what epidemiology was invented for. The origins of the discipline lay in the work of people whom we would now call social scientists: William Petty, William Farr and William Guy in England, the Marquis de Condorcet and Louis Villermé in France, Rudolf Virchow in Germany, and Joaquín Villalba, who coined the name *epidemiología* for the field in 1802, in Spain.[5] These men were interested

4 '121 Cities Mortality Reporting System', available on the CDC website at www.cdc.gov/epo/dphsi/121hist.htm (viewed 18 July 2006).
5 Nancy Krieger recounts some of this history in 'Epidemiology and the social sciences: towards a critical reengagement in the 21st century', *Epidemiologic Reviews*, vol. 22, 2000, 155–63.

in applying quantitative assessments of disease occurrence and vital data to discern how to reshape society so as to make citizens healthier. In contrast, epidemiologists nowadays spend much more time and energy studying how people *behave*.

Behavioural epidemiology

Today is the heyday of behavioural epidemiology. Eat too much and you can become obese. Smoke and you raise your chances of dying of cancer. Have sex without a condom and you might die of AIDS. Life seems thick with risk, some of it still waiting to be detected by a passing epidemiologist. What did you eat for breakfast? Do you buckle up?

An important reason for this shift has to do with a change in what sociologists call the production of scientific knowledge. While the industry of epidemiology strives systematically, scientifically, to generate knowledge, it is no longer in order to learn about the social inequities whose capacity to sicken the populace alarmed epidemiology's nineteenth-century inventors. Now the people who generate such knowledge are the activists and advocates, spokespersons for one or another identity group, or oral historians. Knowledge about how economic mechanisms (the minimum wage, pharmaceutical pricing, 'workfare' in lieu of welfare payments, the male–female wage gap) and social structures (good public schools, inte-grated neighbourhoods, adequate childcare) link to the health of the public is more a matter of lore, or speculation, than epidemiology. The ten issues of the *American Journal of Epidemiology*, the premier professional journal in the field, that appeared from July to December 2004 contained exactly five research articles on how such structural determinants relate to population health (of which four concerned the control of communicable disease epidemics). But the same ten issues contained thirty-seven research articles on behavioural disease risk.[6]

Is American epidemiology turning away from its original *raison d'être* in order to join in the pursuit of a new American order in which those inequities, like poverty and housing discrimination, that are easily seen to be causes of health problems, are to be ignored? By persuading people to focus on their own behaviour, are we epidemiologists helping them to turn their attention *away* from the pressing threats to health of the modern era: astronomical unemployment among urban youth, the warehousing of the homeless, the withholding of medical care from a quarter of the US

6 The remaining 62 of the 104 research articles published in that period concerned either methodological problems or analysed the relation between individually measured non-behavioural covariates, such as genetic type or serologic markers, with individually measured outcomes.

population by denying them health insurance, and the neglect of public housing (or not building it at all)?

No epidemiologist can tell you what your risk of disease is, based on your behaviour. The first reason is because, as I mentioned, risk does not apply to individuals but only to populations. If you want to know what you should do for yourself, you should ask your mother, not an epidemiologist. Second, behaviour is inherently idiosyncratic and constantly varying: even if we were to assemble a group of people who all ate a high-fibre diet every day, we could not be sure that that group's colon cancer rate would be a good basis for predicting the risk of colon cancer for any other group of fibre-eaters. Which is exactly why you hear so many conflicting stories about whether or not you are supposed to be eating broccoli and Grape Nuts.

Still, the thrust of epidemiology lately goes towards calculating the risk allegedly associated with particular activities. Most of the people I know who do this sort of work are well-meaning: they genuinely believe that they will help make people's lives better if they can demonstrate that those who drink sparingly live longer than people who drink heavily, that smokers who quit are less likely to die of lung cancer or heart disease than those who continue smoking, and that everybody is better off using condoms. Probably they are right, in many cases: it is almost always true that smokers will be healthier and live longer if they quit. Epidemiology is valuable because it points the way to reducing disease by modifying the factors that make disease more likely. But what my colleagues do not realize is that their work also supports the delivery of health-risk-avoidance messages to the public in terms that are heavily moralistic. Their work contributes, albeit indirectly, to a new set of pariahs in our society: smokers, women who drink coffee while pregnant, unhelmeted motorcyclists, people who have 'unprotected' sex. So, while it is true for most people that not smoking is better than smoking, and doubtless safer to wear a helmet if riding a motorcycle fast, I must emphasize that epidemiology has very little to say about whether *you* will be better off if you engage in these 'safe' behaviors. Or any individual. Epidemiology can tell you what is likely to happen, but you must understand that that is only a guide, based on the assumption that you are very similar to other people, and that it is always more likely that the predicted event—injury, illness—will not happen to you than that it will. Perhaps the echoes of old-fashioned race accusation are audible in these new moral messages, and in the ostracism that results when people ignore them.

Epidemics and race

In the era of the industrial revolution, cholera was epidemic in the crowded cities of England and the United States. There were 52,000 deaths in England in the 1848–9 epidemic,[7] with as many as 1 or 2 per cent of the population in some impoverished riverside neighbourhoods dying in just a few months. In New York City, cholera killed over 5,000 in 1849.[8] Both liberal social reformers and Christian moralists of the day used the disaster of epidemic cholera to promote the causal metaphor of *miasma*: spumes of decayed organic matter allegedly spreading fearsome diseases to people who lived where there were garbage dumps, cesspools and crowds of unwashed bodies. In both London and New York, many of the indigent were Irish. Attributing the cholera epidemic to miasma was a way of saying: *if only the poor would keep cleaner; if only they would stop drinking so much alcohol; if only they would have fewer babies* ... The myths of the day about Catholics in general and the Irish in particular were wrapped up in the miasma theory.[9] It was the logic of victim-blaming: the Irish poor were responsible for their own decimation; they were responsible not because of how economic necessity forced them to live but because of how they acted; and they were responsible not because of how they really acted but because of how the Irish people as a group were rumoured to act.

In other settings where nationality, religion or skin colour was invoked to explain disease disasters, pretty much the same thing happened. The leading killer throughout the nineteenth century was tuberculosis (TB). Here, too, the effects of social structure were displaced on to behaviour, and behaviour was used to define, and then indict, a race. TB is transmitted by the only unavoidable and unmodifiable activity of life, breathing. It is the classic example of a disease whose distribution is determined purely by social conditions. TB incidence is highest where habitations are most crowded and the nutritional supply is the poorest. Unsurprisingly, it was the leading killer among tenement dwellers in the industrial revolution era, and it remains dangerous to the poor in densely populated places everywhere today.

In the United States before the Civil War, TB was responsible for 20 per cent or more of all deaths, and was more pernicious in the industrial cities of the North than in the still agrarian South. But, exactly because of its high profile, TB could also be turned against American Blacks. Proponents of slavery seized on the North–South difference in TB mortality rates as evidence that the southern way of life was salutary and, in particular, cited the lower rate among slaves compared to Northern Blacks as evidence that black people were a race apart: the

---

7 Sheldon Watts, *Epidemics and History: Disease, Power and Imperialism* (New Haven, CT and London: Yale University Press 1999), 198.

8 John Duffy, *A History of Public Health in New York City 1625–1866* (New York: Russell Sage 1968).

9 This argument is put forth, with a slightly different assessment of its place in the development of a moral agenda in public health, by Charles Rosenberg in *The Cholera Years*, rev. edn (Chicago: University of Chicago Press 1987), see esp. chs 7 and 8.

predisposition of the African American towards TB could be contained only through the benign paternalism of slavery.[10]

Urban TB rates increased further in the later 1800s, as industrialization intensified, immigration expanded and more of the poor crowded into already teeming cities. As Georgina Feldberg shows in her superb book, *Disease and Class*, the prevailing response to TB emerged from Jeffersonian prejudices: Americans held the city *per se* responsible for the high disease rates experienced by its inhabitants.[11] Absent the allegedly salubrious effects of fresh air and the morally uplifting access to agrarian labour and outdoor exercise, the thinking went, city dwellers succumbed to illness. Southern writers focused on the imagined licentiousness of city life as tending especially to raise the risk of TB for black people, whom they imagined to be hereditarily extra-susceptible to consumption.

Of course, removing the shackles from black men and women was dangerous in the southern view, even outside of cities. For instance, the chief medical officer of Mississippi, Dr Henry Rose Carter, definitively asserted that Blacks had brought yellow fever to the United States from Africa and continued to spread it when they were allowed to travel and intermix.[12] The belief that people of African descent were both congenitally resistant to yellow fever (and malaria, another mosquito-borne infection that was a common epidemic problem in nineteenth-century port cities) but ready carriers of those diseases turned race into a catch-22: southern Whites used their conviction that black people were constitutionally resistant to infection to justify assigning black men to work on mosquito-infested docks or in swampland.[13] Naturally, the workers did contract the diseases in such settings. The consequent high rates of disease among the black population validated, for Whites, their assumption that black skin betrayed racial inferiority, notwithstanding the earlier assumption of resistance. And it let white Southerners blame black people's behaviour for transmitting yellow fever and malaria to Whites. Even as they held that black susceptibility to disease was a matter of racial predestination, Southerners argued that the *behaviour* of the black man had to be controlled in order to prevent disease spread.

In our own time, higher rates of both AIDS and heart disease among black Americans have been attributed to habits: African-American AIDS is imputed to the higher number of sexual partners that Black survey respondents admit to, compared to white respondents, to drug injection (although the vast majority of American heroin and cocaine users are white),

10 Georgina Feldberg, *Disease and Class. Tuberculosis and the Shaping of Modern North American Society* (New Brunswick, NJ: Rutgers University Press 1995), 19–35.

11 Ibid., 29.

12 Andrew Spielman and Michael D'Antonio, *Mosquito. A Natural History of Our Most Persistent and Deadly Foe* (New York: Hyperion 2001), 64.

13 Watts, *Epidemics and History*, 215.

and to a rumoured propensity for anal sex. Heart disease is supposedly a function of diet, or an eating 'culture' that disdains low-fat foods, or hip-hop advertising campaigns by McDonalds. Here, too, culpability is fixed by holding African Americans responsible for mythic behaviour: sexual abandon, sexual deviance, primitive eating and dancing rituals, the blood rites of syringe sharing. *If only they could control themselves ...*

In each of these cases, the victims of disease were seen as having brought it on themselves, through some activity rumoured to be characteristic of their group. Aspersions cast on behaviour are magnified by linking the behaviour to a fearsome disease. And the disease thereby helps to identify people as members of the reprobate group. Double whammy: if you are Irish you must drink too much and have too many babies and you are contributing to the spread of cholera; if you get cholera you must be Irish.

The unspoken predicate of the race accusation—the *then* to follow all those *if only*'s—has always been that we would *all* be healthier. Disease culpability takes the accusation that the victims are responsible, through their behaviour, for their own malaise and expands it into a reason for discrimination: *they* are responsible, it says, for *our* malaise, too. So it is nowadays when we accuse young and dark-complected city dwellers of self-destructive (and, usually, immoral) behaviour associated with sex and drug use. It is really an allegation of antisocial intent: society is damaged by the unhealthy activities of 'those people'. The distance between 'us' and 'them' is highlighted by their supposed indiscretions. It makes them a group apart, a race. And while it incriminates them, it exonerates us. The distinction between the members of the inferior race, with their disparaged and harmful habits, and us innocents—the ones *without* race—helps us to identify the implicated.[14] And it allows us to feel that we are 'innocent' victims.

Epidemiology and evolution

I believe that implicating people in the harming of society, through the allegation that their behaviour causes widespread disease, and imagining that people's behaviour expresses their place in a purported hierarchy of races are two harmful forces in public health. And they have much in common, not least an especial historical concurrence. Evolutionary theory and epidemiology appeared at the same historical moment and virtually in a single place. The London Epidemiologic Society was founded in 1850. In 1855 English physician John Snow illustrated the application of the mathematical methods of epidemiology to studying the cause of disease in

---

14 I have drawn the terminology of 'implicated' from Richard Goldstein's 1987 article about AIDS in the *Village Voice*, and his 1988 article in *Milbank Quarterly*, titled 'The implicated and the immune'.

his definitive 1855 second edition of *On the Mode of Communication of Cholera*.[15] Darwin's *The Origin of Species* appeared in 1859.

The link between epidemiology and evolution was forged almost immediately. The new principle of natural selection seemed to make sense of the differential disease occurrence that the also-new science of epidemiology discerned: as higher disease rates were observed among certain peoples—the Irish in England, Africans and their descendents in the United States—the inference that those people were less fit, obviously lower orders of life, seemed validated. In my view, it was not Spencer's 'survival-of-the-fittest' take on evolution or its social Darwinian spawn that led people to look at race categories as pseudo-species, with a self-evident higher class (Protestant Whites) and equally self-evident lower classes. That hierarchy already existed in the minds of people who saw disease as the product of the iniquitous activities of people whom they despised, usually the poor and dark. What the mid-nineteenth-century coincidence of evolutionary and epidemiologic theory did was to legitimate the perception that differential disease rates revealed an intrinsic—that is, biological—social ordering.

Consider tuberculosis again. Once Darwinian theory had come to enjoy wide acceptance in science and after the causative organism of TB had been isolated by Robert Koch in Berlin in 1882, an evolution-inspired definition of race explicitly entered the tuberculosis picture. The American view shifted to what Feldberg calls the 'seed-and-soil' approach: granted TB is triggered by a bacillus, but the disease only develops if the bacterial seed falls on fertile ground.[16] And one of the leading reasons for imagined 'fertility' to TB was evolution: Blacks were held to be uniquely, hereditarily susceptible as a people. As a race, that is. If you think that higher disease susceptibility is an expression of lesser fitness, then you can place the susceptible group—the people at *high risk*, to use modern terminology—lower on the evolutionary ladder.

In the case of yellow fever and malaria, evolution solidified the slavery-era contention that black Americans were uniquely susceptible to disease, and seemed to provide a reason for the lesser fitness that white Americans imputed to black people.[17] Ronald Ross, who claimed to have discovered how malaria was transmitted, wrote while in Sierra Leone that 'the native is ... nearer a monkey than a man'.[18] To Ross and like thinkers, what

15 The full text of Snow's book, as well as maps and statistics on cholera in nineteenth-century London, can be found at Ralph R. Frerichs's encyclopaedic website on Snow, at www.ph.ucla.edu/epi/snow.html (viewed 18 July 2006).

16 Feldberg, *Disease and Class*, 42–8.

17 Watts, *Epidemics and History*, 241.

18 Ibid., 256, quoted from Gordon Harrison, *Mosquitoes, Malaria and Man: A History of Hostilities since 1880* (New York: Dutton 1978), 94. Watts says that Ross was not the discoverer of Anopheles mosquitoes as the vector of malaria; Ross took credit for the work of his assistant Muhammed Bux.

American physicians came to call *diathesis*, a mysterious predisposition to disease, arose because Africans were phylogenetically retarded.

Translating a genetic explanation for disease susceptibility into facile racial accusations sometimes has extreme results, as anyone knows who is familiar with the Nazi euthanasia programme that murdered over 70,000 'Aryan', that is, non-Jewish, Germans beginning in 1939. For our purposes here, what is most significant about the German euthanasia programme is why it ended: it was subsumed, in 1941, within the larger-scale extermination of Slavs, Jews, Gypsies and other *lebensunwerten Lebens*, 'worthless life', the racial offenders who, according to the Nazis, were polluting the German *Volk*. As Götz Aly and colleagues explain in their disturbing book *Cleansing the Fatherland*, the euthanasia programme originally was aimed at reducing the German population's susceptibility to disease and dysfunction by extirpating the genetically compromised.[19] But eliminating the socially dangerous gene turned out to be exactly the metaphor needed to rationalize the Nazis' Final Solution to the race problem. I do not mean to suggest that genetic thinking will make such exterminations happen again. But I do see genetic determinism as a modern version of the seed-and-soil metaphor, continuing to influence how people view disease and having clear links to race. Today, our health officials do not talk about 'worthless life'. But they do connect hereditary disease susceptibility to race when they assert that people of African descent are especially susceptible to specific illnesses.

The diseases to which black Americans are supposedly 'predisposed', or 'at higher risk' of contracting,[20] include such widely disparate conditions as heart disease and stroke,[21] hypertension,[22] prostate cancer,[23] asthma,[24] hepatitis B[25] and HIV infections,[26] infant mortality,[27] and low birthweight,[28] to name only a few. We do know what causes hepatitis B infection, and I

19 Götz Aly, Peter Chroust and Christian Pross, *Cleansing the Fatherland. Nazi Medicine and Racial Hygiene*, trans. from the German by Belinda Cooper (Baltimore: Johns Hopkins University Press 1994), 39, 23 and 44ff.

20 See, for example, the homepage of the Office of Minority Health at the CDC, available at www.cdc.gov/omh/AboutUs/disparities.htm (viewed 18 July 2006).

21 US National Center for Health Statistics (NCHS), *Health, United States, 2005*, Tables 36 and 37, available at www.cdc.gov/nchs/data/hus/hus05.pdf (viewed 19 July 2006).

22 Ibid., Table 69.

23 Ibid., Table 53.

24 NCHS, 'Asthma prevalence, health care use and mortality, 2002', available at www.cdc.gov/nchs/products/pubs/pubd/hestats/asthma/asthma.htm (viewed 19 July 2006).

25 Charles Marwick and Mike Mitka, 'Debate revived on hepatitis B vaccine value', *Journal of the American Medical Association*, vol. 282, no. 1, 1999, 15–17.

26 NCHS, *Health, United States, 2005*, Tables 42 and 52.

27 G. K. Singh and S. M. Yu, 'Infant mortality in the United States: trends, differentials, and projections, 1950 through 2010', *American Journal of Public Health*, vol. 85, 1995, 957–64. See also NCHS *Health, United States, 2005*, Table 20.

28 NCHS, *Health, Unites States, 2005*, Tables 13 and 14.

surmise that it is more common in African Americans for reasons that have to do solely with social clustering: a kind of founder effect—in which the people most likely to acquire an infection and most likely to pass it on are those who are socially linked to the individuals who first contracted the infection—tends to sequestre and amplify sexually transmitted and needle-borne infections like hepatitis B within small social groups. But we do not know completely what the causes are of asthma, prostate cancer, low birthweight or a myriad of other conditions. Claiming that African Americans are predisposed to such conditions explicitly attributes disease risk to genetics and implicitly attributes fitness to race.

Race as metaphor

Metaphors for disease risk, like miasma or seed-and-soil, reinforce popular notions of who is better and who is worse. I see three reasons why genetic determinism is a particularly persuasive metaphor when it comes to explaining disease differences. First, genes do seem to explain some diseases quite well. Tay Sachs, haemophilia and thalassaemia remind us of that. Second, and more perversely, genes seem to offer a biological mechanism by which to justify all those suspicions about racially programmed behaviour and risk, and it is a mechanism that does not require that we mention 'race' at all. And third, genetic determinism allows for very simple explanations about cause.

As for the first reason, the recent finding of differences between 'European' and 'African' populations in the prevalence of a gene that confers prostate cancer risk[29] was widely publicized as implying that it explained Black–White differences in prostate cancer rates.[30] However, a close look at the data reveals that the gene that is reportedly twice as common among the sample of 'African' men in the study than among the 'European' men is found in only 8 per cent of prostate cancer cases. When it comes to pancreatic cancer, stroke, low birthweight or the many other conditions whose occurrence is said to be characterized by racial 'disparity' (to use the term of art), the genetic background that causes these conditions to occur is not clear and simple. Here, and with most conditions, the alleged race correlation of disease occurrence invokes the second and third reasons. And it is the latter, the propensity to adopt simple causal explanations that concerns me here.

29 Laufey T. Amundadottir, Patrick Sulem, Julius Gudmundsson, Agnes Helgason, Adam Baker et al., 'A common variant associated with prostate cancer in European and African populations' (letter), Nature Genetics (online), 7 May 2006 (print publication in vol. 38, no. 6, June 2006).
30 See, for instance, Nicholas Wade, 'Scientists discover gene linked to higher rates of prostate cancer', New York Times, 8 May 2006.

When we say we do not entirely know what causes pancreatic cancer, stroke or low birthweight but that black people are at higher risk, we are saying that we are ready to accept a particular simple causal narrative. Whether we call it 'heredity', 'race' or 'ethnicity', we are saying that something about those people confers differential susceptibility. That simple narrative of cause and effect lets our critical political faculties off the hook. When we accept such simple explanations for disease occurrence we are saying that we do not deem it necessary, as part of the pursuit of better public welfare, to examine the structure of our social arrangements or the economic policies that decree that some people's lives will be straitened and austere while others will live luxuriously. We are saying that we can attribute the higher susceptibility to the things that make *those* people different from *our* people. We do not have to fix the housing, provide the health insurance or reopen the clinics. The problem is in the genes. There is nothing to be done.

Both the epidemiologist's model and that of the geneticist take on extra power when translated into today's science-permeated culture. The modern-day epidemiologist insists that behaviour underlies disease statistics, the molecular biologist ascribes all variation in nature to genes, and the two views together strengthen the race lens through which Americans examine their own culture today.

This lens is a weak one. Even if it had no other faults, the race viewpoint would be suspect because it makes invisible to us the economic constraints—the effects of wealth and social status—that really and irresistibly worsen the public's health. Presumably, many forms of social stratification—not least economic wherewithal—underlie differences in disease rates; to encapsulate in the simple term 'race' the rich explanation of disease rates offered by complex social differences is simplistic. Further, if our desire is to find and then modify the real determinants of disease, the race lens is also beside the point.

It is a dangerous lens to use, too. Constructs like 'race' freight scientific theories with socially volatile cargo. The end result is to disconnect science from the political agendas and social aims that undergird it. The explosiveness of the race issue forces scientists to take cover in an easy pretense of 'objectivity'. When scientists pretend to be objective, they reinforce science consumers' prejudice that scientific findings are specialized knowledge. And when science is thus reduced to a specialty craft that is carried out in isolation from the ebb and flow of social life, political and economic goals seem disconnected from scientific means.

Given the metaphors about risk and race that epidemiology and evolution have inadvertently provided, people who do not want to face up to the tasks of solving social problems and altering the economic policies that contribute to the disease rates in the first place have some convenient options. They can seek to explain why some diseases are more common in some groups of people and less common in others by assigning the cause to genetics.

Increasingly—especially with what Troy Duster calls the 're-biologization of race' through racial interpretations of human genomics findings[31]—attributing causation to genetics means attributing it to race. Those who claim that differences in disease rates are caused by racial differences in the genome can add credibility to their assertions by using the language of biology and evolution. Besides concretizing the concept of 'race' in a genetically-caused-disease foundation, it is a view that absolves its holders of any responsibility to act.

Or (the other option), in the crazy interconnection of morality and morbidity by which our society explains to itself why some people die and others live, the cause of disease can be assigned to individual behaviour. Identifying behavioural causes of disease produces more investment in yet more campaigns to get people to alter their behaviour and live the healthy life. And that allows us, as a society, to continue to ignore the social problems, economic policies and other forms of social stratification that underlie differences in disease susceptibility.

Race is, often enough, where these two options converge. 'Race' is one of the names we give to discontinuities in disease rates. In the United States, 'race' is often the name we give to such discontinuities when they really come from class. In general, the race allegation refers to deficits in wealth or access to power. But it also, nowadays, resonates with assumptions about fitness. You are part of a race if you are identifiable as a member of the *lesser* classes, not just of the lower strata economically, but of the groups whose disease rates are higher.

We can say that the differences we observe in disease rates arise from genetics, or we can say that the differences arise from engaging in improper behaviour. But in either case what we mean is that those people—the ones who are 'at higher risk', the ones who are 'hereditarily' susceptible—are the *loci* of disease. They carry risk in their genes. They are socially suspect. They are implicated. And since we are innocent, we do not have to solve, or necessarily even examine, the vexing problems of modern society that truly make some people sick while others are well.

Philip Alcabes, an epidemiologist, is Associate Professor in the School of Health Sciences, Hunter College of the City University of New York. He has published numerous research articles on AIDS and other social-epidemiologic problems, which have been the subject of his work since the early 1980s. He also writes and lectures on epidemiology and ethics, and public policy aspects of disease control.

31 Troy Duster, 'Buried alive: the concept of race in science', *Chronicle of Higher Education*, 14 September 2001, B11–12.

The molecular reinscription of race: unanticipated issues in biotechnology and forensic science

TROY DUSTER

ABSTRACT   In the last five years, there has been a considerable increase in the number of published articles documenting the health disparities between the majority white population and various other racially designated groups in the United States. This was a direct result of the congressional mandate given to the National Institutes of Health in 2000 to conduct research and report findings on the topic. It was inevitable that reports of patterned disparities between racially designated groups would resuscitate an old debate about whether there were important biological differences between such groups. There is now a new role in this debate for biotechnology firms committed to finding markets for pharmaceutical products that have failed to get past clinical trials aimed at the general population. By refocusing marketing strategy on racially designated populations, the industry has gathered support for medicines that were previously 'racially neutral'. And this strategy has in turn inspired 'strange bedfellow' support from clinicians who claim selective advantage for their patients from such 'racialized medicine'. There has been a parallel development in forensic science. There are new claims that DNA analysis of crime scene data will assist criminal investigations by narrowing the search for suspects along racial lines. Because these tests are privately conducted, it is not possible for critics to assess the sampling procedure or the overall methodology that is used in categorizing human populations by race. Nonetheless, these claims dovetail with those in pharmacogenomics that assert the importance of patterns in the DNA for 'predicting' ethnic and racial membership. In sum, these developments are ushering in an era of the molecular reinscription of race in the biological sciences.

No one could have predicted that the Defense Department's commissioning of a secure high-speed communication network for military use would 'spin off' into the World Wide Web of the contemporary Internet. While the Defense Department achieved its goal, that achievement has been dwarfed by the scale of the social, economic and political consequences of the way the Internet has developed. From daily commercial transactions to downloads of streaming videos, from distance learning to search engines that can mine the Library of Congress, from e-mail to news media clips to blogs, the list could go on for several pages. The Internet is such a dominant feature of the lives of so many that, on a worldwide scale, if banks or hotels or restaurants do not have their own websites, they are consigned to outlier status in the backwaters of an integrated global network. No one could have predicted the speed and penetration of these developments. But, if we had stopped and thought about it, we might have expected dramatic changes if the known synergistic ingredients to the infrastructure were to be placed on to the conveyor belt of modern life.

In a parallel fashion, one of the deeply consequential spin-offs of the mapping and sequencing of the entire human genome has been the use of these technologies to identify individuals at the level of the microchip. This capacity for the identification of millions, even billions, across the globe is going to produce spin-offs that will ultimately dwarf the original intentions of the early advocates of a genome map. The first of those is just now emerging: the subtle, sometimes inadvertent, reinscription of race at the molecular level. A second development—the use of markers for individual identification and for claims to 'authenticity' of group membership—has already penetrated deep into the criminal justice system by way of forensic applications. This includes the use of DNA in post-conviction cases to determine whether there has been a wrongful conviction, the kind of situation that might result in freeing the innocent. Another use involves the collection of DNA from suspects or arrestees in pretrial circumstances to increase the DNA database, which in turn is designed to help law enforcement officers find matches between the DNA samples of those suspects or arrestees and tissue samples left at some unsolved crime scene: a net to catch the guilty. This is a long way from the original reason for mapping the genome.

The rationale behind the Human Genome Project, and for the Haplotype Map Project that followed,[1] has always been the search for ways to improve health.[2] There have already been some health benefits, and there will certainly be more. Nonetheless, in this essay I will point to mounting evidence that the inadvertent and unintended spin-offs (into domains far removed from health concerns and clinical medical applications) of the revolution in human molecular biology will dwarf the medical achievements.

In the last five years, there has been a peculiar and fateful irony in the convergence of the desire (and pressure) to use genetics to improve our health, and the decision by the US Congress to require that the National Institutes of Health record data and engage in research to lessen the health disparities between racial and ethnic groups. In 2000 Congress passed the Minority Health and Health Disparities Research and Education Act of 2000

1 International HapMap Consortium, 'The International HapMap Project', *Nature*, vol. 426, 18 December 2003, 789–96.
2 The rationale for the Icelandic database, for the Howard University database and for the Estonian database is also in each case explicitly about strategies for improving health.

(Public Law 106-525), which mandated the National Institutes of Health to support research on health disparities between groups categorized by race and ethnicity.

As a direct consequence, the years since have seen a sharp increase in the number of articles that report health disparities between members of the majority white population and the various groups racially and ethnically designated. That was to be expected. Moreover, since the National Human Genome Research Institute is a branch of the National Institutes of Health, it would follow that research on human genetics would enter the fray, with scientists poised and ready to assert the unique contribution of molecular genetic differences to an explanation of these health disparities. For example, because the rate of prostate cancer in African Americans is more than double that in white Americans, it was inevitable that some would attempt to explain this through the lens of genetics. This in turn would lead the way to rescuing old racial taxonomies and their relationship to genetic profiles and genetic conditions. It was not expected that this strategy would thereby inadvertently resuscitate the idea that genetic differences between those we place in racial categories might well explain different health outcomes. This is territory full of minefields for obvious reasons that date back to the eugenics movement in the United States and its promulgation and extension into Nazi Germany.[3]

To navigate around such problems, research scientists have developed two strategies. The first is to use only an *ex post facto* deployment of race and ethnicity, after data have been collected in large clinical trials in which 'race' had not been a defining category of selection. Two recent examples of this are the marketing of the racialized drugs BiDil (for relief of hypertension and congestive heart failure amelioration in African Americans) and Iressa (a drug for treatment of late-stage lung cancer in Asians). The second strategy for avoiding the explosive combination of race-genetics-disease is to propose a large-scale research project aimed at determining the genetic *v.* environmental causes of health problems. Of course this proposal presumes that one can successfully disentangle the genetic from the environmental. It is one of the most fundamental axioms of contemporary life sciences that there is an interactional element at the core of the relationship between genes and environment. To assert that some human health condition, trait or behaviour is, say, 60 per cent genetic and 40 per cent environmental is to express a static and archaic version: a statistical artefact of the static assumption.[4] Such a

3 Philip R. Reilly, *The Surgical Solution: A History of Involuntary Sterilization in the United States* (Baltimore: Johns Hopkins University Press 1991); Stefan Kühl, *The Nazi Connection: Eugenics, American Racism, and German National Socialism* (Oxford and New York: Oxford University Press 1994); Robert N. Proctor, *The Nazi War on Cancer* (Princeton, NJ: Princeton University Press 1999).

4 Richard C. Lewontin, 'Analysis of variance and analysis of causes', *American Journal of Human Genetics*, vol. 26, no. 3, 1974, 400–11.

statistical 'parcelling out' denies or obscures the profoundly interactional relationship between race, genes and disease, now generating one of the most vexing and visceral debates in contemporary science. In order to understand why, we must first try to understand what it means to 'isolate' 'race' as a variable (or constant) in a research protocol. The first part of this essay addresses the subtle reinscription into the biological sciences and clinical medicine of an old notion, pre-dating molecular biology, of human taxonomies of race. The second part follows on from a discussion of the population-specific DNA databases to address their forensic use as markers for identification.

Navigating with (and around) race

Biotechnology firms have found an unusual and effective way around the problem of confronting 'race' as a 'biological category'. Their strategy is *not* to deal with race by means of a full-scale, case-control research design, but to 'back into' a clinical study that was never designed to test whether race played any role only to discover *ex post facto* that the race of the clinical population, however defined, *did* play a role in drug efficacy. The reinterpretation by racial categories of already collected data sets conveniently circumnavigates the problem of having to define terms. After all, to do a case-control study would require the researcher to define terms and to specify the boundaries of the relevant populations. For 'race', this would be a knotty problem these days when the primary criterion for racial classification is self-reporting.

BiDil and the medicalization of the sources of hypertension

BiDil is a combination of isosorbide dinitrate and hydralazine designed to restore low or depleted nitric oxide levels in the blood to treat or prevent cases of congestive heart failure. It was originally designed for a wide population base; race was irrelevant. But the early clinical studies revealed no compelling results, and a Food and Drug Administration (FDA) advisory panel voted 9 to 3 against approval.

In a remarkable turn of fate, however, BiDil was suddenly born again as a racialized intervention. One of the investigators went back into the data, and found that African Americans in the original clinical trial seemed to fare better than Whites. Because the study was not designed to test that hypothesis, a new clinical trial would have to be approved. However, rather than setting up a study designed to see whether BiDil worked better in one group than in another, in March 2001 the FDA approved a full-scale clinical trial, the first to be conducted exclusively in black men and women suffering from heart failure.

The BiDil Blacks-only trial reflects two problematic assumptions about race and medicine. The first is that African Americans' risk of developing and dying from heart failure is twice that of Whites. This claim has been floating around in the scientific literature for more than a decade, mainly uncontested. Jonathan Kahn recently completed some remarkable scientific sleuthing on the topic, however, and showed that the claim by NitroMed, the company that developed BiDil, about the scale of Black–White difference is simply untrue. Kahn traced the citation sources back nearly two decades, and demonstrated conclusively that the difference between Blacks and Whites is actually closer to 1.2:1.[5] There is a difference, but it is nowhere near the 2:1 ratio that would warrant special trials for one population group. Thus, a substantial section of the scaffolding of the BiDil clinical trial is built on incorrect statistical data about racial disparities. The second claim is that BiDil has a special effect that is greater in African Americans than in Whites.[6] The clinical trials were not designed to test that hypothesis. Rather, by concentrating only on Blacks, the study can have little or nothing compelling to say about comparative results, by race.

In the early spring of 2005, anticipating the FDA decision to approve the drug in late spring, NitroMed released a statement that was an attempt to provide a justification for the approval of the drug as race-specific: 'The African American community is affected at a greater frequency by heart failure than the corresponding Caucasian population. African Americans between the ages of 45 and 64 are 2.5 times more likely to die from heart failure than Caucasians in the same age range.'[7] The figures are technically correct, but the age-group 45–64 only accounts for about 6 per cent of heart failure mortality, while those over 65 constitute 93.7 per cent of the mortality. Moreover, over 65, the statistical differences between 'African Americans' and 'Caucasians' almost completely disappear. Why the focus on race? What is at stake and why is NitroMed so invested in selectively portraying these sharp racial differences? Part of the answer lies in the role of prospective markets for biotech products. While the new mantra of biotechnology is the claim that pharmaceuticals will someday soon be marketed to individuals based on their DNA, the fundamental truth is that selling drugs is about markets. These markets are not about individual designer drugs, but about groups and population aggregates that become target markets.

5 Jonathan Kahn, 'How a drug becomes "ethnic": law, commerce, and the production of racial categories in medicine', *Yale Journal of Health Policy, Law, and Ethics*, vol. 4, no. 1, Winter 2004, 1–46.
6 Anne L. Taylor, Susan Ziesche, Clyde Yancy, Peter Carson *et al.*, 'Combination of isosorbide dinitrate and hydralazine in Blacks with heart failure', *New England Journal of Medicine*, vol. 351, no. 20, 11 November 2004, 2049–57.
7 NitroMed press release, 'FDA accepts NitroMed's new drug application resubmission for BiDil', 2 February 2005, available at http://investors.nitromed.com/phoenix.zhtml?c = 130535&p = irol-newsArticle&ID = 670434&highlight = (viewed 8 August 2006).

The original BiDil patent was not race-specific, but it expires in 2007. By making the drug race-specific, the patent will be extended another thirteen years to 2020. This gives NitroMed the exclusive right to market the drug as a therapy for heart conditions. This whole process has succeeded in biologizing and medicalizing 'race' in ways that could have been easily avoided ... if market forces were not dominating the decision-making. By simply testing generic drug combinations of hydralazine and isosorbide dinitrate in comparison populations, the question of drug efficacy would have been answered. But such a strategy would have undermined the marketing monopoly and would have, instead, brought relatively cheap drugs to the market. This strategy would have 'saved lives' in a more comprehensive and race-neutral way, in sharp contrast to the rhetoric being deployed by those marketing BiDil, who say that, regardless of the socio-political aspects of marketing a drug that is race-specific, the drug 'saves lives'.

In a classic piece of epidemiological research, Michael Klag and his associates showed a decade ago that, in general, the darker the skin colour, the higher the rate of hypertension for American Blacks, even within the African American community.[8] Klag *et al.* indicated that this was not biological or genetic in origin, but biological in effect, due to stress-related outcomes of reduced access to valued social goods such as employment, promotion, housing and so on. The effect was biological, not the cause.

Iressa, lung cancer and Asians

The British/Swedish firm AstraZeneca conducted a large clinical trial across the full population of patients suffering from advanced stages of lung cancer to test the efficacy of Iressa, one of its most promising drugs. The drug was first introduced in 2002, and over 45,000 patients worldwide have taken it. It is designed to treat the most common form of lung cancer by blocking an enzyme that otherwise causes cancer cells to proliferate. In the full study, the difference between those on placebo and those taking Iressa was statistically insignificant. When the results were announced, the FDA began reviewing the situation to determine whether the drug should be pulled from the market. However, in viewing the data by race and ethnicity, it was determined that, while the average number of months that life was prolonged was 5.5 for the general population, Asians had a 9.5-month prolongation, nearly twice as long. Immediately, AstraZeneca touted the findings as significant, and began preparations for shifting their marketing strategies and sales to Asian countries.[9]

8 Michael Klag, P. K. Whelton, J. Coresh, C. E. Grim and L. H. Kuller, 'The association of skin color with blood pressure in US Blacks with low socioeconomic status', *Journal of the American Medical Association*, vol. 265, no. 5, February 1991, 599–602.
9 Nicholas Zamiska and Jeanne Whalen, 'Cancer drug, deemed failure, helps Asians', *Wall Street Journal*, 5 May 2005, B1.

Two elements have now combined in a synergistic way to set the stage for the 'hurricane just offshore' that is waiting for the winds to change. The first concerns the new diagnostic technologies of bio-informatics, computer-assisted analyses of patterns of DNA. The second concerns new research on specific populations and allele-frequency markers for those populations that just happen occasionally to coincide with the socially defined groupings we used to call 'ethnic' or 'racial', but are now increasingly referred to as groups aggregated by 'population-specific allelic frequency patterns'. With the latest computers, we can now put the DNA of several clusters of people on computer chips, and see what patterns in their DNA might emerge.

We can perform hundreds, even thousands, of such experiments in a few hours. Sometimes this proves to be a useful technology in the hunt for particular regions in order to help explain some illnesses. For example, if we get a few hundred patients, all with prostate cancer, then we can look for patterns in their SNP profiles using the chip technology.[10] With the new SNP profiles, it is possible for a researcher—by simply sorting those affected, and not driven by any theoretical question—to come up with new taxonomies of people who share certain patterns in their DNA. That is the way much of clinical genetics tries to find 'candidate genes' for a particular condition, say, prostate cancer, among those who suffer from it. But what happens when rates of prostate cancer differ significantly between groups that have been racially designated? This way of framing the problem leaves one vulnerable to making a profoundly subtle interpretive error, namely, that, by holding other factors constant statistically (such as income, education, class etc.) and finding persistent racial differences, one has substantial grounds for concluding that race is more biological than social and political. The following example provides an illustration of how this error is made, both in the natural sciences and the social sciences.

The interpretive error: controlling for other factors and the biology of race

In 1986 the Drug Enforcement Administration initiated Operation Pipeline, a programme designed in Washington, D.C. that ultimately trained 27,000 law enforcement officers in forty-eight participating states over the ensuing decade. The project was designed to alert police and other law enforcement officials as to the 'likely profiles' of those who should be stopped and searched for possible drug violations. High on the list were young, male African Americans and Latinos driving in cars that sent signals

10 Single nucleotide polymorphisms (SNPs) are DNA sequence variations that occur when a single nucleotide (A, T, C or G) in the genome sequence differs between members of a species (or between paired chromosomes in an individual). For example a SNP might change the DNA sequence AAGGCTAA to ATGGCTAA. SNPs make up about 90 per cent of all human genetic variation.

that something might be amiss. For example, a nineteen-year-old African American driving a new Lexus would sound an 'obvious' alarm because the assumption is that the family could not afford such a car, and that the driver must therefore be 'into drugs'. In a study of the I-95 highway corridor just outside of Baltimore, police records indicated that Latinos and Blacks were eight times more likely to be stopped by the police than Whites.[11] A young white male in his early twenties driving a Lexus would not be considered 'suspicious', since the police are more likely to assume that he is driving the family car. So, if class is statistically held constant, and a racial difference is still found, it would be a massive interpretive error to conclude that, since race is still a factor, it must be operating as a biological variable. The same would be true for the study of a medical condition, say, hypertension. If the researcher has statistically controlled for social class and race still shows up as a risk factor, it does not mean that the social meaning of 'race' is not present. Middle-class African Americans are subject to more stressors than middle-class Whites, and that is a social reality that may have biological outcomes, not origins.[12]

The segue to forensics, criminal justice and 'molecular race'

It is possible to make arbitrary groupings of populations—defined by geography, language, self-identified faiths, other-identified physiognomy and so on—and still find statistically significant allelic variations between those groupings. For example, we could simply pick all of the people in Chicago, and all of the people in Los Angeles, and find statistically significant differences in allele frequency at *some* loci. Of course, at many loci, even most loci, we would not find statistically significant differences. When researchers claim to be able to assign people to groups based on allele frequency at a certain number of loci, they have chosen loci that show differences between the groups they are trying to distinguish.

The work of Ian Evett *et al.*, Alex Lowe *et al.* and others suggests that only about 10 per cent of DNA sites are 'useful' for making distinctions.[13] This

---

11 Troy Duster, 'Selective arrests, an ever-expanding DNA forensic database, and the specter of an early twenty-first century equivalent of phrenology', in David Lazer (ed.), *DNA and the Criminal Justice System: The Technology of Justice* (Cambridge, MA: MIT Press 2004), 315–34.

12 Raymond Franklin, *Shadows of Race and Class* (Minneapolis: University of Minnesota Press 1991).

13 I. W. Evett, J. S. Buckleton, A. Raymond and H. Roberts, 'The evidential value of DNA profiles', *Journal of the Forensic Science Society*, vol. 33, no. 4, 1993, 243–4; I. W. Evett, P. D. Gill, J. K. Scranage and B. S. Weir, 'Establishing the robustness of Short-Tandem-Repeat statistics for forensic application', *American Journal of Human Genetics*, vol. 58, 1996, 398–407; Alex L. Lowe, Andrew Urquhart, Lindsey A. Foreman and Ian W. Evett, 'Inferring ethnic origin by means of an STR profile', *Forensic Science International*, vol. 119, no. 1, 2001, 17–22.

means that, at the other 90 per cent of the sites, the allele frequencies do not vary between groups such as 'Afro-Caribbean people in England' and 'Scottish people in England'. But it does not follow that, because we cannot find a single site at which allele frequency matches some phenotype—we are trying to make identifications for forensic purposes, we should be reminded—there are not several (four, six, seven) sites that could be effective in aiding the FBI, Scotland Yard or the criminal justice systems around the globe in formulating highly probable profiles of suspects, and the likely ethnic, racial or cultural populations in which they can be found … statistically.

So, when molecular biologists assert that 'race has no validity as a scientific concept', this is apparently in contradistinction to the practical applicability of research on allele frequencies in specific populations. It is possible to sort out and make sense of this—and even to explain and resolve the apparent contradiction—but only if we keep in mind the difference between using a taxonomic system with sharp, discrete, definitively bounded categories, and one that shows only patterns (with some overlap) but that may prove to be empirically or practically useful.

When representative spokespersons from the biological sciences say that 'there is no such thing as race', they mean, correctly, that there are no discrete racial categories that come to a discrete beginning and end, that there is nothing mutually exclusive about our current (or past) categories of 'race', and that there is more genetic variation within categories of 'race' than between them. All this is true. However, when Scotland Yard or the Birmingham police force or the New York Police Department wants to narrow the list of suspects in a crime, they are not primarily concerned with tight taxonomic systems of classification with no overlapping categories. That is the stuff of theoretical physics and philosophical logic, not the practical stuff of crime-solving or the practical application of molecular genetics for health delivery via genetic screening, and all the messy overlapping categories that will inevitably be involved with such enterprises. That is, some African Americans have cystic fibrosis even though the likelihood of that is far greater among Americans of North European descent and, in a parallel if not symmetrical way, some American Whites have sickle cell anaemia even though the likelihood of that is far greater among Americans of West African descent. But in the world of cost-effective decision-making, genetic screening for these disorders is routinely based on commonsense versions of the phenotype. The same is true with regard to the quite practical matter of naming suspects.

In an article in the 8 July 1995 issue of *New Scientist* entitled 'Genes in Black and White',[14] some extraordinary claims are made about what it is possible to learn about socially defined categories of 'race' from reviewing information

14 Gail Vines, 'Genes in black and white', *New Scientist*, no. 1985, 8 July 1995.

gathered using new molecular genetic technology. In 1993 a British forensic scientist published what is perhaps the first DNA test explicitly acknowledged to provide 'intelligence information' along 'ethnic' lines for 'investigators of unsolved crimes'.[15] Ian Evett, of the Home Office's forensic science laboratory in Birmingham, and his colleagues in the Metropolitan Police claimed that their DNA test could distinguish between 'Caucasians' and 'Afro-Caribbeans' in nearly 85 per cent of cases. Evett's work, published in the *Journal of the Forensic Science Society*, draws on apparent genetic differences in three sections of human DNA. Like most stretches of human DNA used for forensic typing, each of these three regions differs widely from person to person, irrespective of race. But, by looking at all three, the researchers claimed that under select circumstances it was possible to estimate the probability that someone belonged to a particular racial group. The implications of this for determining, for practical purposes, who is and who is not 'officially' a member of some racial or ethnic category are profound.

The legal and social applications of these technologies are already in considerable use by the *cognoscenti*, and they are poised to 'take off' even further. For example, more than a decade ago, several states began keeping DNA database files on sexual offenders. Three factors converged to make this a popular decision by criminal justice officials and one that would be backed by politicians and the public: 1) sex offenders are those most likely to leave bodily tissue and fluids at the crime scene; 2) they rank among the most likely repeat offenders; and 3) their crimes are often particularly reprehensible in that they violate persons, from rape to molestation and abuse of the young and most vulnerable. Today, all fifty states store DNA samples of sex offenders, and most states do the same for convicted murderers. However, thirty-four states now store DNA samples of all felons.[16] Since 1 September 1999, the state of Louisiana has taken a DNA sample of all those merely arrested for a felony.[17] In compliance with its 1998 state law, Virginia now has a website listing its registered sex offenders, a practice[18] followed by Indiana, Florida and Alaska. So, what started off as concern with sexual offences has now widened to include many other felonies.

15 Ian W. Evett, 'Criminalistics: the future of expertise', *Journal of the Forensic Science Society*, vol. 33, no. 3, 1993, 173–8.
16 Tania Simoncelli, 'Dangerous excursions: the case against expanding forensic DNA databases to innocent persons', *Journal of Law, Medicine and Ethics*, vol. 34, no. 2, 2006, 390–7.
17 Paul E. Tracy and Vincent Morgan, 'Big Brother and his science kit: DNA databases for 21st century crime control', *Journal of Criminal Law and Criminology*, vol. 90, no. 2, 2000, 635–90 (682).
18 See the 'Sex offenders and crimes against minors registry' on the Virginia State Police website at http://sex-offender.vsp.virginia.gov/sor/index.htm (viewed 16 August 2006).

Function creep: from Social Security to DNA databanks

Social Security in the United States was originally intended only as a federal retirement programme. The entire scheme was vigorously debated in the 1930s, and some members of Congress argued vehemently that the Social Security identification card should not be a national identification card. The vote in the Congress was close. However, the Internal Revenue Service (IRS) soon began using the Social Security number to track citizens for tax-collection purposes. It was later used by many public services as a required personal identification number and, still later, private institutions began to demand it for identification purposes. This process is called 'function creep': the process by which the original function may remain, but newer uses expand into ever-widening spheres.

Since it is the state that is primarily involved in criminal law enforcement, there have been state-by-state variations in the use of DNA databanks and storage. Fifteen years ago, most states were only collecting DNA samples from sexual offenders. Now, seven states require the DNA databanking of *all* felons, including those involved in white-collar felonies. When Governor Pataki proposed such a scheme for New York state, the state legislature forced him to jettison the idea. Louisiana was the first state to pass a law mandating the collection of DNA samples from anyone arrested for a felony but, in the past five years, it has been joined by Virginia and several other states. That is, just like 'function creep' with regard to Social Security identification numbers, the use by states of DNA databanks is rapidly expanding.

Today, thirty-eight states store samples from varying categories of lawbreakers in a DNA databank. Twenty-nine states now require that tissue samples be retained in their DNA databanks after profiling is complete.[19] Only one state, Wisconsin, requires the destruction of tissue samples once profiling is complete. What started as a tool for dealing with sex offenders has now 'crept' into a way to deal with lawbreakers and those merely arrested.

While thirty-nine states permit the expunging of samples if charges are dropped, almost all of those states place the burden of initiating the destruction of samples on the individual. Thus, civil privacy protection, which in the default position places the burden on the state, is reversed. With the reauthorization of the 2005 Violence against Women Act, the burden for expunging samples shifts to the individual who has been placed in the federal CODIS (Combined DNA Index System) database.

19 Jonathan Kimmelman, 'Risking ethical insolvency: a survey of trends in criminal DNA databanking', *Journal of Law, Medicine and Ethics*, vol. 28, no. 3, 2000, 209–21 (211).

Twenty states authorize the use of databanks for research on forensic techniques. Based on the statutory language in several of those states, this could easily mean assaying genes or loci that contain predictive information, even though current usage is restricted to analysing portions of the DNA that are only useful as identifying markers. Since most states retain the full DNA (and every cell contains all the DNA information), it is a small step to using these DNA banks for other purposes. The original purpose has long been pushed to the background, and the 'creep' extends not only to crimes other than sexual offenses, but to misdemeanours and even arrestees.

On 5 January 2006, the President of the United States signed into law HR 3402, the Department of Justice Reauthorization of the Violence against Women Act of 2005. For the first time this legislation gives state and federal law enforcement officials the right to enter DNA profiles of those merely arrested for federal crimes into the CODIS database. Previously, only convicted felons could be included. Those DNA profiles will remain in the database unless and until those individuals who are exonerated or never charged with the crime request that their DNA be expunged. Thus the default position will be to store these profiles, and expunging requires the proactive agency of those arrested. This announcement was a cause for celebration by one of the leading providers of DNS testing services, Orchid Cellmark, Inc., of Princeton, New Jersey. The president and chief executive officer of Cellmark, Paul J. Kelly, immediately issued a statement applauding this development, stating:

> This is landmark legislation that we believe has the potential to greatly expand the utility of DNA testing to help prevent as well as solve crime … It has been shown that many perpetrators of minor offenses graduate to more violent crimes, and we believe that this new legislation is a critical step in further harnessing the power of DNA to apprehend criminals much sooner and far more effectively than is possible today.[20]

Britain has been in the vanguard of these developments, but there is every indication that this will not be so for long.[21] In April 2004 a law was passed in the United Kingdom permitting police to retain samples from anyone arrested for any reason, including people who are not charged with a crime.

---

20 'Orchid Cellmark hails passage of landmark legislation expanding use of forensic DNA identity testing in the U.S.', press release, 6 January 2006, available at www.orchid.com/news/view_pr.asp?ID = 393 (viewed 17 August 2006).

21 The British may be in the lead, but the Portuguese have even bigger plans: in early April 2005, the Portuguese government announced that it intended to collect DNA on all of its residents, all of its inhabitants. Maria João Boavida, 'Portugal plans a forensic genetic database of its entire population', *Newropeans Magazine* (online journal), 8 April 2005, at www.newropeans-magazine.org/index.php?option = com_content&task = view&id = 2059&Itemid = 121 (viewed 17 August 2006).

Anyone can have their DNA taken and stored. The database already contains 2.8 million DNA 'fingerprints' taken from identified suspects, plus another 230,000 from unidentified samples collected from crime scenes.[22] Samples are being added at the rate of between 10,000 and 20,000 per month.[23] The aim is to have on file a quarter of the adult population's DNA, a figure that exceeds ten million, making it by far the largest DNA database in the world. In keeping with the 'racialization' of DNA forensic databases, it was recently disclosed that nearly 4 in 10 Blacks are in the UK forensic database, compared with fewer than 1 in 10 Whites.[24] Perhaps the most striking statistic comes from the fact that police record 'the ethnic appearance' of each person placed in the database: 82 per cent of male profiles are white, while only 7 per cent are black, according to the Home Office. Thus, comparing the proportion of each racial grouping in the database against their proportion of the whole population reveals the sharp disparity. Because many of these individuals are involved only in arrests, civil libertarians have wondered out loud about the implications for the presumption of innocence. Dominic Bascombe, a writer for a London-based newspaper (*The Voice*), expressed his concern that these data reflected the greater likelihood that Blacks face arrest: 'It is simply presuming if you are black you are going to be guilty—if not now but in the future.' He then noted that this constituted what he called 'genetic surveillance' of Blacks: 'We certainly don't think it reflects criminality.'[25] 'Anyone in the database—and family members—can more easily be linked to a crime scene if their DNA is found there. This may be because they are a criminal, or because they visited the scene prior to the crime.'[26]

The New York Police Department, with the urging and support of Mayor Rudolph Giuliani, was chafing to make use of a portable DNA lab kit.[27] At the time this was being proposed, in 2000, New York Police Chief Howard Safir said that a DNA sample should be taken from 'anyone who is arrested for anything'.[28] This lab kit, the convergence of molecular genetics and contemporary concerns, was developed by the Whitehead Institute for Biomedical Research. By the year 2010 it is likely that we will be using these technologies far more in relation to forensics and the law than to medicine and therapies. California passed a ballot proposition in 2004 that permits, by

22 'Police aim for DNA on 25% of UK population', *British Journal of Healthcare Computing & Information Magazine*, February 2005, abstract at www.bjhc.co.uk/news/1/2005/n502020.htm (accessed 17 August 2006).
23 And this was before the bombings in London on 7 July 2005.
24 James Randerson, 'DNA of 37% of black men held by police', *Guardian*, 5 January 2006, 1.
25 Quoted in Randerson, 'DNA of 37% of black men held by police'.
26 Randerson, 'DNA of 37% of black men held by police'.
27 Ayana Mathis, 'Stop, drop, and swab: New York police ponder portable DNA labs', *Village Voice*, 6 June 2000, 26.
28 Tracy and Morgan, 'Big Brother and his science kit', 665.

2008, the collection and storage of DNA data not only on all felons, but on arrestees and those committing some categories of misdemeanours.

New York state collects fingerprints from persons receiving public assistance (to prevent duplicate claims) and has done so since 1994, but does not generally share those data with law enforcement. In that state, the record of one's arrest must be sealed, and employers cannot ask if someone has ever been arrested. However, an employer can ask if someone has been convicted. When a mere arrest triggers DNA sampling and storage, when those samples are not expunged, the record becomes analogous to radioactive storage in that it keeps emitting its effect indefinitely.[29]

Population-wide DNA databases

It is now relatively common for scholars to acknowledge the considerable, and documented, racial and ethnic bias in police procedures, prosecutorial discretion, jury selection and sentencing practices, in which racial profiling is but the tip of an iceberg.[30] Indeed, racial disparities penetrate the whole system and are diffused throughout it, all the way up to the racial disparities involved in seeking the death penalty. If the DNA database primarily includes those who have been touched by the criminal justice system, and that system operates practices that routinely select more from one group than another, there will be an obvious skew or bias towards this group. Some have argued that the way to handle the racial bias in the DNA database is to include everyone.

But this does not address the far more fundamental problem of the bias that generates the configuration and content of the criminal (or suspect) database. If the lens of the criminal justice system is focused almost entirely on one part of the population for a certain kind of activity (drug-related street crime), and ignores a parallel kind of crime (fraternity cocaine sales a few miles away), then, even if the fraternity members' DNA is in the databank, they will not be subject to the same level of matching or of subsequent allele frequency profiling research to 'help explain' their behaviour. *That behaviour will not have been recorded.* That is, if the police are not arresting the fraternity members, it does not matter whether their DNA is in a national database because they are not *criminalized* by the selective targeting of the criminal justice system.

Thus, it is imperative that we separate arguments about bias in the criminal justice system at the point of contact with select parts of the population, from 'solutions' to bias about 'cold hits'. It is certainly true that, if a member of the fraternity committed a rape, left tissue samples at the scene and—because he was in a national DNA database—was nabbed by the

29 Kimmelman, 'Risking ethical insolvency'.
30 Marc Mauer, *Race to Incarcerate* (New York: New Press 1999).

police with a 'cold hit', that would be a source of justifiable affirmation. But, by ignoring powder cocaine and emphasizing street sales of cocaine in the African American community, the mark of criminality is thereby generated, and this is not altered by having a population-wide DNA database.

However, the surface fiction of objectivity will lead to a research agenda concerning DNA. There is a serious threat regarding how these new technologies are about to be deployed that is masked by the apparent global objectivity of a population-wide DNA database. I am referring to the prospects for SNP profiling of offenders. As noted, even if everyone were in the national database, this would not deter the impulse to do specific and focused research on the select population that has been convicted.

Troy Duster is Director of the Institute for the History of the Production of Knowledge and Silver Professor of Sociology at New York University. His most recent books are *Backdoor to Eugenics* (2nd edn, 2003) and (with Michael K. Brown *et al.*) *Whitewashing Race: The Myth of a Colorblind Society* (2003).

Biobanks of a 'racial kind': mining for difference in the new genetics

SANDRA SOO-JIN LEE

ABSTRACT   While social scientists have argued that race emerges through a historically grounded context and is best understood as fluid and reactive to historical and political conditions, genetics and the search for differences revisit notions of race as embedded in the physical body. Lee argues that DNA repositories maintain both physical and symbolic space for notions of genetic essence among human groups whereby 'race' is framed as a natural kind. She argues that, despite rhetorical strategies to de-race the new genomics, the ongoing significance of racial differences in the naming of groups reveals the socio-cultural context in which genomic science is produced and translated into clinical medical practice. In addressing the seeming paradox between the *mantra of sameness*, which emphasizes that humans share 99.9 per cent of their genetic material, and the current infrastructure of biobanks being built in support of research on difference, Lee examines three DNA banks and discusses the emergence of the trope of 'genetic particularity'. She argues that this trope is possible through a reframing of the human genome as not one collective, common blueprint, but rather as derivations of a theme whereby diversity is translated into 'racial identity' relinked to biological difference.

Herein lie buried many things which if read with patience may show the strange meaning of being black here in the dawning of the Twentieth century. This meaning is not without interest to you, Gentle Reader; for the problem of the Twentieth Century is the problem of the color-line.

—W. E. B. Du Bois, *Souls of Black Folks* (1903)

In the introduction to his treatise on race relations in the United States, W. E. B. Du Bois forewarned that the 'color-line' would emerge as the central social challenge shaping the contours of group relations. His words proved prescient not only for the twentieth century and may be even more relevant in the present, at the dawn of the twenty-first. While discourse on race has proliferated in the public sphere, it has done little to interfere with the ongoing search for difference in defining where and how the color-line should be drawn. Critical to this endeavour has been the use of 'technologies of racialization' in highlighting, demarcating and exacting difference from the human body, and translating skin tone, eye shape and blood type into proxies for group identity. The recent surge in human genetics research through the development of high-throughput technologies and the decipher-ing of the genomic alphabet into meaningful categories of risk is the latest to be deployed in 'race-making', in which the colour-line is inscribed beyond the surface of the skin. Although the scientific community has repeatedly affirmed that the vast majority of the human genome is synonymous among human beings, a growing chorus of scientists contends that the key to understanding the genetic basis of disease and variability in drug response lies in the minute difference between groups.[1] This has fuelled the hunt for variation in the single base pair mutations known as single nucleotide polymorphisms, or SNPs, that are estimated to occur once in every thousand base pairs,[2] and can vary in frequency among populations. Such efforts coincide and in some cases have prompted the creation of national biobanks that catalogue human DNA samples that will be mined for genetic difference. This has resulted in the creation of a biobanking infrastructure that places in stark relief the shifting and contingent meanings of national, 'racial' and ethnic identity in the new genetics, and begs closer examination of their effects on trajectories of enquiry and their implications for under-standings of social identity and difference.

This essay examines the ways in which cell repositories construct race through human genetic variation panels and provide the architecture for research on population differences. In the title of the essay, I suggest that DNA databases may be compared to 'biobanks of a kind'. In this discussion, I engage the Aristotelian notion of 'kinds' as those entities that are understood by their 'essences'. As such, 'kinds' are believed to have their own intrinsic reality, apart from the particular circumstances in which they are discovered. While social scientists have argued that race emerges through a historically grounded context and is best understood as fluid and reactive to historical and political conditions, genetics and the search for differences revisits notions of 'race' as embedded in the physical body. Treated as material reality, race is recast as a natural kind while, at the same

---

1 The 'common disease–common variant' hypothesis suggests that common diseases such as coronary heart disease, diabetes and certain types of mental illnesses are associated with genetic variants that are relatively frequent in most human populations. A competing theory is that such diseases are associated with several different rare variants, which would not be captured by the current approach of mapping common variants through large-scale projects such as the International HapMap Project to be discussed below.

2 SNPs are those base pair differences that are often identified as mutations. For example, one individual may have a nucleic acid base of G (guanine) where another individual has one of C (cytosine).

time, understood as a by-product of the social world. Philosopher Naomi Zack addresses this apparent paradox and writes: 'Again, the genes for traits deemed racial are scientifically real but, there is no racial aspect of these genes which is scientifically real. And yet, on a folk level the prevailing assumption is that race itself is physically real.'[3] Race becomes embedded in the body through a slippage whereby traits and conditions that travel with race become understood as artefacts of race itself. Sickle cell anaemia is a good example of the racialization of disease. Keith Wailoo, in his detailed study, shows how this illness becomes inextricable from 'blackness' and a narrative of racial biology sets off a trajectory of public health policy that embeds race into algorithms of susceptibility and risk.[4]

By suggesting that genomics beckons the notion of 'race' as naturalized by genes, the body becomes the ground in, from and on which racial difference can be discovered, excavated and held up for inspection. The identification of 'kinds' reveals taxonomies of difference or systems in which a classificatory schema creates order through a logic that comes with the mere act of sorting things.[5] This essay argues that DNA repositories maintain both physical and symbolic space for notions of genetic essence among human groups whereby 'race', framed as a natural kind, forces further consideration of the production of human identity through the assemblage and classification of human genetic materials into national biobanks. Despite rhetorical strategies to de-race the new genomics, the ongoing significance of racial differences in the naming of groups reveals the socio-cultural context in which genomic science is produced and translated into clinical medical practice. In addressing the seeming paradox between the *mantra of sameness*, which emphasizes that humans share 99.9 per cent of their genetic material, and the current infrastructure of biobanks being built in support of research on difference, I examine three DNA banks and the effort to create distinctive national repositories. By drawing on these examples of biobanking, I discuss the emergence of the trope of 'genetic particularity' that insists on a framework of race whereby meaningful biological differences lie waiting to be 'read' from individual genetic codes. This trope is possible through a reframing of the human genome as not one collective, common blueprint, but rather derivations of a theme whereby diversity is translated into 'racial identity' relinked to biological difference. This notion of genetic particularity provides the justification for the creation of the ever-growing DNA biobanks

3 Naomi Zack, *Thinking about Race* (Belmont, CA: Wadsworth Publishing 1998), 54.
4 Keith Wailoo, *Dying in the City of the Blues: Sickle Cell Anemia and the Politics of Race and Health* (Chapel Hill: University of North Carolina Press 2001); Melbourne Tapper, *In the Blood: Sickle Cell Anemia and the Politics of Race* (Philadelphia: University of Pennsylvania Press 1999).
5 Geoffrey C. Bowker and Susan Leigh Star, *Sorting Things Out: Classification and Its Consequences* (Cambridge, MA and London: MIT Press 1999).

in the United States and elsewhere, further entrenching the 'racial' dimension to human genetic variation research.

   This essay focuses on the creation of DNA repositories in Iceland, South Korea and the United States, and is part of an ongoing study of the meanings of 'race' in the context of emerging genomic technologies and their use in biomedicine.[6] Using my background in anthropology and ethnographic approaches, I attempt to understand the often competing perspectives of social actors on the relationship between genes, race and human identity: how they emerge within a set of institutional arrangements and how such constraints impact on the type of decisions that can be made in human genetic variation research. My research methodologies include in-depth interviews conducted with geneticists, bioethics specialists, policymakers, social scientists, community representatives as well as other stakeholders in the identification, storage and distribution of genetic samples in national biobanks. This study is also a result of archival research and participant observation of associated meeting, workshops, conferences and forums about policies on categorizing and storing DNA samples and the taxonomies used to characterize human genetic variation. A central goal of the research is to discover how the creation of biobanks both informs and impacts on social knowledge of the human body and on what constitutes meaningful human difference.

The paradox of race in the new genetics

Despite the increasing focus on recent developments in human genetics, the seemingly simple question of what is a 'gene' remains a challenge to answer. Even molecular biologists use multiple definitions of what counts as genes. While genes are understood to be made up of DNA and DNA's nucleic acids are understood to be the human hereditary units that determine human physiology, which 'parts' of DNA should be counted as the gene is far from being a straightforward issue. While scientists argue over the significance of RNA molecules and 'coding' and 'noncoding' regions, what becomes clear is that, as Evelyn Fox Keller has noted: 'The very meaning of any DNA sequence is relational—for the purpose of understanding development or disease, the patterns of genetic expression are what really matter ... and they cannot be predicted from knowledge of the sequence alone.'[7] The gene forms only when DNA is put in a meaningful context.

---

6 'The ethics of identifying race in the new genetics', National Human Genome Research Institute, National Research Service Award, September 2000–July 2003, Ethical, Legal and Social Implications Program, no. F32HG000221.
7 Evelyn Fox Keller, 'The century beyond the gene', *Journal of Biosciences*, vol. 30, no. 1, February 2005, 3–10 (4).

What I call the 'new genetics' may be ushering in an era in which the pendulum swings back to conceptions of 'race' based on biology. The new genetics, as described by Kaja Finkler, refers to knowledge and procedures derived from DNA technology that bring 'into the forefront of people's consciousness the genes carried by individuals and their families'.[8] In the compression of time and space, the new genetics forges a consciousness among groups of a genetic basis for common heritage and lineage. Identifying such linkages may allow the new genetics to have profound effects in the field of medicine, particularly for the discovery of 'risk' and for raising hopes for the greater understanding and ultimate control of genetically inherited diseases and adverse drug response. The new genetics has been compared to a new medical toolbox whose use will result in new boundaries between healthy and unhealthy people, and risk factors being uncovered before the onset of physical indications of disease.

The new genetics grows out of the confluence of developments in technology and the gathering belief that genes will provide clues to the most common and deadly of diseases. Strides in biocomputing that have simultaneously hugely increased the speed by which data may be processed allowed the completion of the Human Genome Project (HGP), a hallmark event of the new genetics, to occur ahead of schedule in 2003 and, perhaps more remarkably, under the proposed budget of $300 million.[9] The public and private venture of the HGP, funded by the National Human Genome Research Institute (NHGRI) of the National Institutes of Health (NIH) and the Celera Genomics Corporation, a private genome company, resulted in an unprecedented sharing of research data and made possible the sequencing of the three million base pairs that make up the human genome. The HGP was pivotal in defining the era of the new genetics because of its scale but also in giving rise to an implicit promise that research on genes would yield clues to defining who is, and what it means to be, human.

On the question of race, the message that resulted from the completion of the HGP was unified and clear: race was not to be found in the genome. In a White House press conference on the project's completion in June 2000, President Clinton stated:

> After all, I believe one of the great truths to emerge from this triumphant expedition inside the human genome is that in genetic terms all human beings, regardless of race, are more than 99.9% the same. What that means is that modern

8 Kaja Finkler, *Experiencing the New Genetics: Family and Kinship on the Medical Frontier* (Philadelphia: University of Pennsylvania Press 2000), 3.
9 Total expenditure for the duration of the Human Genome Project from 1993 to 2001 amounted to approximately 264 million.

science has confirmed what we first learned from ancient faiths. The most important fact of life on this Earth is our common humanity.[10]

His conclusions were echoed by Francis Collins, Director of the NHGRI, who expressed awe at the 'first glimpse of our own instruction book, previously known only to God'. Collins stated definitively that the only 'race' one could speak of was the 'human race'.[11] This was reiterated by Craig Venter, then President and Chief Scientific Officer of Celera, who explained that, after sequencing 'three females and two males who have identified themselves as Hispanic, Asian, Caucasian or African-American' and were included 'out of respect for the diversity that is America', he could comfortably conclude that 'the concept of race has no genetic or scientific basis'.[12]

Despite the fanfare associated with these proclamations, they were hardly newsworthy. Prior research in human population genetics had reached the same conclusion in the previous several decades and the debate over the biological basis for race was largely believed to have been 'won' by those who emphasized its *social construction* and pointed to the historical mutability of what has counted as 'race' in the United States. Several professional organizations, including the American Sociological Association and the American Anthropological Association, issued statements before the completion of the HGP disputing the use of 'race' as a biological variable and emphasizing the concept of 'ethnicity' as a more useful term that addressed the social and cultural factors inherent in group identity. The American Association of Physical Anthropologists in their 'Statement on the Biological Aspects of Race' had proclaimed: 'There is great genetic diversity within all human populations. Pure races, in the sense of genetically homogenous [*sic*] populations, do not exist in the human species today, nor is there any evidence that they have ever existed in the past.'[13] The near mantra-like statements of 'sameness' made by the architects of the HGP—that there is more genetic variability *within* populations than *between* them—were already familiar through the earlier work of population geneticists,[14] and confirmed what most social and life scientists seemed to have already accepted: race is not genetic.

It is thus with some irony that, now, a mere three years after the momentous celebration of the HGP's conclusion, the current trajectory of genomic research is increasingly focused on the 0.01 per cent genetic difference that is believed to separate one individual from another. The

---

10 Quoted in 'Reading the book of life: White House remarks on decoding of genome', *New York Times*, 27 June 2000.

11 Ibid.

12 Ibid.

13 'AAPA statement on the biological aspects of race', *American Journal of Physical Anthropology*, vol. 101, 1996, 714.

14 Richard C. Lewontin, *Biology as Ideology: The Doctrine of DNA* (New York: Harper Perennial 2001).

search for functional genetic variability is increasingly taken up in populations that are identified by conventional notions of 'race'. This trajectory is
the result of a confluence of factors, including a growing infrastructure of
research materials that are racially categorized through the creation of
biobanks. Such sorting practices reflect the ongoing conflict over the
meaning of 'race' in science and medicine. In the emerging era of the new
genetics, in which super-computer technology has given way to an explosion
of human genetic data, biobanks that utilize taxonomies of race in the
classification, storage and distribution of DNA samples become 'racializing
technologies' that promote notions of racial biology in research protocols
designed to discover group difference.

Biobanks and the re-emergence of the 'kind'

Naomi Zack, in her interrogation of the materializing of race as a 'kind', has
outlined the 'one-drop rule' that has been used historically to define
'blackness' in the United States. She describes a schema in which an
individual, S, is black if S has one black forebear any number of generations
back; an individual, Y, is white if Y has no black forebears any number of
generations back (and no other non-white forebears). Zack explains that this
classificatory system was intended to signify that the categories of 'black'
and 'white' were mutually exclusive. In the same way, genomics research
and technology make claims for such demarcations. What is often lost but
must be remembered is that the identification of SNPs is always a function of
numbers. The notion that populations carry with them unique, signature
mutations is, of course, a misunderstanding. Identifying difference is an
inherently subjective endeavour in which relative frequencies reflect overlapping patterns, and differences are measured through statistical algorithms rather than the presence or absence of specific SNPs. Despite the
consistent message from population geneticists that difference should be
understood in terms of *clinal variation*, and that variation occurs in degrees
without sharp boundaries between groups, 'race' as a by-product of genetic
particularity persists as the predominant trope of human difference. In the
new genetics, the biological basis for race continues to loom large in the
public consciousness despite the widely publicized conclusion of the HGP
that denies its genetic validity. Taxonomies used in the classification of DNA
for biobanking become an instrumental technology for racialization whereby
relative frequencies of difference are recast within categories that imply
group boundaries.

Current gene sequencing and data mining projects have resulted in the
near frenzied international search for functionally significant SNPs. This has
served as the impetus for national initiatives for repositories in Iceland, the
United Kingdom, Japan, China, Estonia and other countries in which
national identity and the donation of genetic samples combine to form a

narrative of particularity and primordial identity that privileges ideas of historically uninterrupted lineage as the bedrock for contemporary social identity. Primordialism is evident in the Icelandic biobank, created by deCODE Genetics, which, according to the company's description, was founded on an extensive genealogy database that includes over 680,000 records, 'covering more than half of all the Icelanders who ever lived'.[15] The database attempted to chronicle virtually all Icelanders who were born in the nineteenth and twentieth century as well as most individuals from the eighteenth century. Cast as a living archive and a tribute to Iceland's past, the database is called the 'Book of Icelanders' after the *Íslendingabók*, the earliest preserved book of Icelandic history that was written around 1130 by 'Ari Þorgilsson the Learned'. Citing a high rate of inclusivity, the company argues that it has an explicit advantage over other such biobanks in pursuing links between genes, disease and drugs. The company states:

> The Book of Icelanders includes more than 95% of all those who have lived in Iceland since the first nationwide census in 1703, and stretches back to the first settlers in the 9th century. In total, it includes over 680,000 entries, recording more than half of all Icelanders who have ever lived. The database is also extraordinarily accurate. deCODE has analyzed its accuracy using genotypic data and has established that, even after accounting for laboratory error, *the connections in the genealogies are more than 98% correct*.[16]

While deCODE's difficulties in achieving its desired level of participation are well known, this company statement reflects the salience of perceived accuracy of lineage for researchers interested in finding genetic clues to phenotypes in question. What is left unstated but presumed is the premium placed on 'purity' in identifying the Icelandic database as a national biobank. The assertion of Icelandic particularity is achieved through a coupling of breadth (asserted by the high rate of inclusion of the current Icelandic population) and depth (claims that the bank reaches back to the original settler population). As such, the company emphasizes that virtually all individual genomes have been historically accounted for and that the biobank is an enclosed and whole system. Individual samples are thus linked as part of a shared collective in which national boundaries are intertwined with DNA. The collection is envisioned as a unique entity unto itself: its intrinsic worth is derived less from the individual genomes sampled than from the aggregated whole that has been characterized as Iceland, the nation-state. It is at the level of population that the biobank will be inspected for its particularity in the hunt for clues to disease and drug response.

15 'The population approach', formerly on the deCODE website at www.decode.com/ Population-Approach.php (no longer available, viewed 10 November 2003).
16 Ibid. (emphasis added).

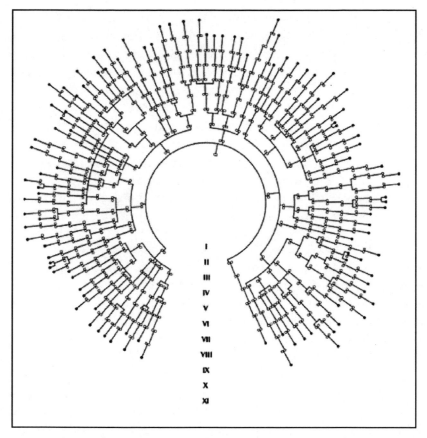

Figure 1   A family tree of 102 Icelandic asthma patients, linked together over eleven generations back to a founder couple born in the mid-seventeenth century.
Source: 'The population approach', available on the deCODE website at www.decode. com/Population-Approach.php (viewed 13 September 2006).

An example of the potential utility of a collection of DNA with known lineage is illustrated in the family tree (see Figure 1). The image depicts 102 Icelandic asthma patients linked together over eleven generations back to a founder couple born in the mid-seventeenth century. The ability to conduct disease/gene association studies may be significantly enhanced through such biobanking efforts. The national biobank may function as an extrapolation of the family tree, casting itself as a set of unique genetic signatures that are linked to one another in functionally significant ways. In this way, the biobank becomes a repository of relatedness that is understood as complete and particular to a given group of people.

The merging of national and genetic identity is certainly not unique to Iceland and can be found in other attempts to create national biobanks. In South Korea, the biotechnology company Macrogen announced its intention to map the 'Korean genome', understood to be different from the human genome already sequenced through collaborative efforts in the United States. In the reporting of the genome project, the Korean daily newspaper *Chosun*

Ilbo justified the project by stating that 'the successful drafting of the [Korean] map follows the announcement of the successful mapping of genomes for *Caucasians* done by Celera Genomic, a US bioengineering company in June of last year'.[17] Contrary to assertions that the HGP was a map applicable to all humans, the Korean genome effort reflects an understanding of the HGP as applicable only to a race of 'Caucasians'. This reading of the HGP map may reflect the chasms that divide genomic science despite its context of increasing globalization. The lingering East/West racial divide is clear in the justification for the Korean genome and emphasizes notions of inherent biological differences.

Similar to the efforts in Iceland, the South Korean company offers its rationale of the project by invoking notions of purity and particularity:

> As Korea has a strong tendency to propagate within its race, Korea maintains a relatively pure blood pool as compared with members of other nations. So, we expect that a study of several participants' genome structure will give us a Korean specific genome structure. This project will also help us to obtain Korean genomic blueprints including patterns of single nucleotide polymorphisms (SNPs). The results of the Korean genome project will be the basis for developing personalized medicine in the near future.[18]

Echoing the claims of the Icelandic biobank, the justification for a separate Korean genetic project is based on beliefs of racial purity and the need to capture genetic 'specificity' unique to the Korean people. The assumption is that without 'Korean genomic blueprints', the anticipated benefits of the new genetics will not materialize. The argument that a national DNA project is essential in order to create 'personalized medicine' reflects the somewhat ironic conflation of individual genomes into a national, yet personalized racial kind that is framed as distinct from other 'racial types' already sequenced. The goal, according to company chairman Suh Jeong-seon, is to 'decode the biological definition of the word "Korean"'.[19] The claim is that in genes resides an elusive essence of Korean identity that is critical to understanding and treating the Korean body. It is in this construction of genes that processes of racialization occur in which difference is understood as both inherent and prescriptive.

17 Cha Byung-hak, 'Bio-tech firm completes draft of Korean genome', *Chosun Ilbo*, 26 June 2001 (emphasis added).
18 Webpage formerly on the Macrogen site describing the Korean genome project, at www.macrogen.com/english/index.html (no longer available, viewed 10 November 2003).
19 'Biotech firm reveals first ethnic Korean genome map', *Korea Now*, 30 June 2001, available at http://kn.koreaherald.co.kr/SITE/data/html_dir/2001/06/30/200106300007.asp (viewed 18 August 2006).

Attempting colour-blindness

The creation of national biobanks is both a material endeavour in which samples of human blood are labelled, stored and ultimately distributed for research, as well as the creation of a critical site for forging social identity. In the cases of Iceland and South Korea, homogeneity and purity were seen as characteristics of Icelandic and Korean identities, and narratives justifying biobanking focused on a singular identity. The creation of a national biobank in the United States forces a somewhat different negotiation of the complex meanings of race, genes and national identity, prompting a struggle over how to characterize genes and the meanings of 'race' in scientific research.

In 1998 the NIH launched an initiative for the large-scale discovery of SNPs, mutations that occur along the human chromosome that may ultimately be of use in the study of disease and drug response. As part of this initiative, the NHGRI created a DNA resource for SNP discovery called the DNA Polymorphism Discovery Resource, or PDR, and placed it in the public domain. The PDR contains the DNA samples and cell lines of 450 anonymous, unrelated US residents of whom there are an equal number of men and women. According to the PDR architects, these samples were taken from individuals who were identified as European-American (including non-Hispanic Whites), African-American (including non-Hispanic Blacks), Asian-American (including individuals with ancestry from East and South Asia) and Mexican-American.[20] Such sampling was conducted as a method of ensuring a broad array of what its creators called the 'genetic representation' of the nation.[21]

Although the NIH went to great lengths to include what its architects believed were samples representative of the diversity that constitutes the United States, the agency took the historic step of excising information on racial and ethnic identity from individual DNA samples. In doing so, the NHGRI attempted to prevent researchers from using such information in their research analysis. Included in the use agreement of the PDR is the following clause: 'Researchers who wish to use the DNA Polymorphism Discovery Resource or the database are required to agree to not try to identify the ethnicity of the samples when they obtain them or access the

20 Francis S. Collins, Lisa D. Brooks and Aravinda Chakravarti, 'A DNA Polymorphism Discovery Resource for research on human genetic variation', *Genome Research*, vol. 8, no. 12, December 1998, 1229–31.
21 Samples of American Indian tribes were not included in the PDR. According to PDR working group members, this decision was made in reaction to previous political controversy over the collection of DNA for research purposes. Details of this decision deserve an extended discussion not possible within the constraints of this essay. I do, however, discuss this issue in a paper on the development of the PDR, 'Racial realism and the struggle over health disparities in a genomic age', in Barbara Koenig and Sandra Soo-Jin Lee (eds), *Revisiting Race in a Genomic Age* (forthcoming from Rutgers University Press).

information in the database.'[22] In the interviews I conducted with indivi-duals associated with the creation of the PDR, this decision to 'de-race' the repository was based mainly on two factors. The first was the explicit and repeated reference to the controversy around the Human Genetic Diversity Project (HGDP) that had attempted to sample globally, including indigenous groups who protested against the project, accusing it of being a form of biocolonialism.[23] In an effort to avoid a similar politicization of the new DNA bank, the PDR architects decided to prevent the repository's samples from being associated with any particular racial group and to try to monitor scientists who might attempt to draw their own conclusions. The second reason for the 'colour-blind' policy stated by the PDR architects was the pressure placed on the NIH by would-be users of the repository in the scientific community to make the resource available immediately. As one PDR working group member put it, the geneticists 'were clamoring for the samples and we couldn't justify the time it would take to think through how to deal with the race issue. The policy we ended up with was a short cut.' By shelving the 'race issue', the PDR working group hoped that it would be side-stepping the political quagmire around race, power and the body that loomed large in the institutional memory of the NIH.

Expediency, the hallmark challenge of the new genetics, was to be balanced against the ethical problem of the 'race issue'. The policy to expunge race from the PDR samples was not a by-product of the belief that race was not salient to genetic research but rather an attempt to circumvent its potential politicization. One working group member summarized the trade-off in this way:

> Policies on how to identify and categorize [human] genetic variation are only half dictated by science. The other half of the equation is public reaction. Ever since the HGDP there has been increasing sensitivity around how best to handle sampling issues ... We were not ready when the resource was established so we decided to table it. We needed to get the samples out but didn't know how yet to deal with the race issue.[24]

The decision to 'get the samples out' illustrates the attempt to decouple the bodily materials from origin, ancestry or identity. This decision assumed that the samples were in their essence the same with or without identifying information. With such materials in hand, the biobank architects expected that science would be allowed to continue its work unimpeded (because race is not genetic) while a policy that addressed the looming socio-political

22 'A DNA Polymorphism Discovery Resource', available on the NHGRI website at www.genome.gov/10001552 (viewed 19 August 2006).
23 See Jenny Reardon, *Race to the Finish: Identity and Governance in an Age of Genomics* (Princeton, NJ and Oxford: Princeton University Press 2005).
24 Interview with a molecular biologist, 5 March 2003.

concerns could be formulated. The presumption was that science functioned separately from the social and that the boundaries between them were discrete and manageable.

An important feature of the PDR was the effort of its architects to represent the diversity of the United States in the inclusion of samples from racially identified populations. While the samples were stripped of this information, they were dispersed to researchers in 'predefined nested subsets with 8, 24, 44, and 90 samples encompassing the same range of diversity as the complete set'.[25] In maintaining a 'balance' of genetic diversity, one may argue that the PDR attempted to 'nationalize' the collection while suppressing the importance of race. However, the colour-blind policy resulted in muted success, attesting to the incontrovertible entanglement of science in the social and society's nagging influence on science. According to interviews with users and potential users, the PDR has become one of the most under-used repositories in the NIH collection and was described by more than one geneticist as 'useless'. During an interview, one such researcher explained this assessment by stating emphatically:

> Look, I am not out to draw racist conclusions in my work. In fact, I don't even do comparative research but *I* want to know. It's part of the subjects who contributed the samples and by trying to strip them of that information, you are left with an incomplete picture. Researchers want to know what they are dealing with.[26]

This geneticist makes plain what perhaps gives rise to the paradox around race. While there is resistance among most to the idea of a biological basis for race, race remains important stock knowledge that provides the contours, however amorphous, of the world in which we work. Scientists, as we well know, are no less informed by these tacit assumptions. Hence, the demand to know 'what they are dealing with' reflects the fact that scientists are deeply enmeshed in a social world where the seamless incorporation of ideas, values and 'truths' of social relationships influence the design and execution of science.

Some scientists argue that little attention is being given to whether race is 'real', and that the controversy over race in science and, in particular, genomics research has become a game of semantics and political rhetoric. They claim the focus is solely on the politically defensible strategic use of terms rather than on open enquiry into the possible connections between

---

25 'DNA Polymorphism Discovery Resource', available on the Coriell Cell Repositories website at http://locus.umdnj.edu/nigms/products/pdr.html (viewed 19 August 2006).
26 Interview with a human geneticist, 25 March 2003.

race and human biology. One genetic epidemiologist questions the point of such efforts, asserting:

> The reality is that the population is segmented and that differences exist ... It might be politically correct to avoid the word 'race', but at some point we need to tackle the hard issues ... that these things matter. In the not so distant future, we are going to see numerous associations and it will not be so easy to take the position that race does not exist.[27]

This scientist's statement is a familiar retort to the argument that race is a mutable category that historically has responded to changing socio-political conditions. As Bruno Latour states in his treatise on the perspectives of scientists:

> If you point out politely that the very ease with which scientists pass from the social world to the world of external realities, the facility they demonstrate through this business of importing and exporting scientific laws, the fluency of the discourse in which they convert human and objective elements, prove clearly enough that there is no rupture between the two worlds and that they are dealing rather with a seamless cloth, you will be accused of relativism; you will be told that you are trying to give Science a 'social explanation' ... [28]

Genomic science is no different in the efforts of its scientists to retain boundaries in the name of pure and unfettered enquiry. The decision to make the PDR colour-blind was to many scientists a case of the NIH pandering to politics instead of revealing what is presumed as scientific truth: that DNA is inextricable from where it originates and the category of scientific analysis is not 'nation' but 'race'.

Entrenching race in biomedical research

While some have claimed that the new genetics will render race obsolete through the discovery of genetic etiologies, current practices reflect a research infrastructure built on the presumption that 'race' is a necessary variable for biomedical research, and further entrench its use in the identification of human genetic materials. Population geneticist Neil Risch has taken the lead in arguing for the use of race in biomedical research into genetic epidemiology. In an article first published in *Genome Biology* entitled

---

27 Interview with a genetic epidemiologist, 8 April 2003.
28 Bruno Latour, *Politics of Nature: How to Bring the Sciences into Democracy*, trans. from the French by Catherine Porter (Cambridge, MA and London: Harvard University Press 2004).

'Categorization of Humans in Biomedical Research: Genes, Race and Disease', Risch *et al.* argue that 'the greatest genetic structure that exists in the human population occurs at the racial level'.[29] The authors build on this claim by making the increasingly commonplace assertion that 'race' will continue to be the best proxy for genetic relatedness in disease association studies until it becomes feasible to do routine whole genome scans on individuals.

A central challenge for those advocating the use of 'race' as a biological variable is identifying a racial taxonomy that draws rational boundaries between populations. This question over who and what constitute racial identities has led to confusion over categorizing practices. Even a cursory review of the taxonomies used by both publicly and privately funded cell repositories reveals a potpourri of terms, including 'nationality', 'ethnicity', 'territory', 'region', 'citizenship' and 'skin colour', as proxies for human genetic variation.[30] Recognizing this, governmental agencies have embraced US Census categories as the best standard of racial classification. Most recently, in January 2003 the Food and Drug Administration (FDA) drafted guidelines to standardize race information, advocating the use of Census categories in the collection of race and ethnicity data in clinical trials under its jurisdiction.[31] In its draft guidance, the FDA does not explain how researchers should go about defining the Census categories, nor does it offer any basis for accepting them as the best standard. Rather, the guidance cites the similar practice of its sister institution, Health and Human Services, emphasizing the need for administrative continuity. This need further embeds race and race-thinking into the research process. Without consensus on the definitions of the Census categories, much less their validity as scientific variables, the move by the FDA in following convention contributes to a trajectory of race-based science.

While the regulatory infrastructure of biomedical research more deeply embeds race into what constitutes relevant science, the argument for racial categories has been further justified by the national public health goal of

29 Neil Risch, Esteban Burchard, Elad Ziv and Hua Tang, 'Categorization of humans in biomedical research: genes, race and disease', *Genome Biology*, vol. 3, no. 7, July 2002, 1–12 (4).

30 For a broad range of DNA collections, it is instructive to review those housed by the Coriell Cell Repositories (CCR) at the Coriell Institute for Medical Research. Located in Camden, NJ, the CCR is funded by the National Institutes of Health and holds the world's largest collection of human cell cultures. The human genetic variation panels established by the National Institute for General Medical Sciences (NIGMS) are a good illustration of the numerous taxonomies used to indicate racial and ethnic differences. See 'Human variation collections of the NIGMS repository', available on the CCR website at http://ccr.coriell.org/nigms/cells/humdiv.html (viewed 23 August 2006).

31 Department of Health and Human Services, Food and Drug Administration, 'Draft guidance for industry on the collection of race and ethnicity data in clinical trials for FDA regulated products', *Federal Register*, vol. 68, no. 20, 30 January 2003, 4788–9.

reducing health disparities between racially identified populations. Citing the significant differences in morbidity and mortality between historically racially identified groups, the NIH set as its goal the elimination of disparities by the year 2010. As a result, all research programmes funded by the NIH must include racially identified individuals in their research protocols. In fact, the burden of identifying human subjects by race in order to satisfy federal requirements meant to ensure 'inclusion' of historically excluded racialized populations falls squarely on the shoulders of researchers, whose funding is placed in jeopardy by failing to monitor and report the racial and ethnic identification of their human subjects. Race, thus, becomes an a priori, yet undefined, *de facto* scientific variable in every research project funded by the NIH. In cyclical fashion, these demands inform policies that ascribe 'race' to DNA samples and the organization of research materials into biobanks. Without requiring researchers to define how race operates in their study protocols, it may be unclear how 'race' is being interpreted: as primarily a social artefact in the study of health disparities and/or the role of environmental factors that may significantly impact on health status, *or* as a proxy for biological difference. The unqualified racial labelling of DNA that strips genes of the life history, social context and experience of those who have donated these bodily materials allows for a pendulum shift in scientific discourse that racializes genes as biologically inherent. These assertions lie in tension with the strong and seemingly unconditional message that genetic differences between groups matter little compared to individual differences within populations.

Race-making through biobanking

On 27 May 2003 the *New York Times* reported that Howard University, a historically black university in Washington, D.C., was planning to create the largest repository in the United States of DNA to be taken from over 25,000 African Americans over a five-year period. The new repository, to be named the Genomic Research of the African Diaspora biobank, or GRAD, would be used in research on identifying genetic contributions to disease and drug response. The *New York Times* ran the story under the headline 'DNA of Blacks to Be Gathered to Fight Illness'. In reporting the new repository, the article included a confusing and somewhat paradoxical quote from a NIH official. Disputing the utility of race in genetics research, the official stated: 'There's 10 times more difference between a white person and his Caucasian wife than between a white population and an African population.' This familiar point echoes the resounding conclusions of the HGP that human beings share 99.9 per cent of their genome with each other. However, he continued his remarks by stating that studies of 'African American genes' could be useful in fighting disease.[32] This recapitulation of the mantra that we are all the same only then to be followed by an unproblematized reference to 'African American genes' is a good example of the current approach in relaying genetics research to the public. The initial 99.9 per cent reference does the work of acknowledging the elephant in the room: namely, that the new genetics must be situated within the greater history of racism and violence that has used genetic science in the subjugation of human groups. The mantra that humans are predominately the same justifies the new genetics and its trajectories of enquiry on difference as somehow decoupled from yesteryear's eugenics. This discursive work is effective for it, paradoxically, allows for the justification of the creation of biobanks in which DNA samples are sorted according to a racial logic that imbues bodies and bodily materials as natural kinds. This logic clears the way for the reification of race and genetic essentialism.

The mantra of sameness is perhaps a uniquely American strategy. Whereas other nations might be less willing to espouse the idea that racially identified individuals are by and large the same and that race is not genetic, American ideals of equity and inclusion spill over into how genomic science is relayed to the public. The incongruity between ideals and what some have called 'scientific truths' has generated controversy over the use of race in human genetic research and in biomedicine. The result is the current mottled landscape of contradictory decisions and policies. For those at the forefront of the new genetics, the colour-blind approach of emphasizing sameness may at first seem effective. However, its execution, as illustrated by the PDR, is fraught with contradiction. The rejection of the PDR colour-blind policy and the institutional use of racial categories in both research and clinical medicine reflect the continued salience of race for scientists. These cultural practices conceal 'race' as a socially constructed category and further reify it as phenomenologically inextricable from the gene.

The shift to 'populational thinking', according to Lisa Gannett,[33] creates a calculus of human qualities that are mapped on to discrete classifications. The effort in South Korea, like Iceland's deCODE database, is part of the new wave of biobanking spawned by the quest for defining and creating such differences in the new genetics. Such national projects have emerged throughout the world, articulated through the rhetoric of national identity, race and biological specificity. However, in the search for common variants causing common diseases such as coronary heart disease, diabetes, depression and other conditions, what type of information can be gleaned from DNA that is presumed to be particular and unique within the global context?

---

32 Andrew Pollack, 'DNA of Blacks to be gathered to fight illness', *New York Times*, 27 May 2003, A1.

33 Lisa Gannett, 'Racism and human genome diversity research: the ethical limits of "populational thinking"', *Philosophy of Science*, vol. 68 (Supplement), September 2001, S479–S492.

Will the discovery of different genetic associations for common diseases challenge our current notion of *human* diseases that affect all populations? Will such notions of particularity challenge definitions of common diseases and result in the emergence of distinct forms, such as Icelandic diabetes or Korean depression? How does an infrastructure of research that presupposes group difference put in motion trajectories of enquiry that recapitulate ideas of distinct groups?

Race has from its inception been a tool for organizing the world: a social tool. In the new genetics, a struggle over identity can occur over how to characterize difference between populations and the meaning of the relative presence and absence of SNPs. Biobanking efforts rely on racial taxonomies in the organization of DNA samples. These sorting practices may have significant implications for upstream research that links disease, drug response and other characteristics to identified groups. The fundamental question is why does 'race' as a natural kind continue to emerge as an attractive concept? Why do we return to such questions, using the latest scientific developments to posit notions of racial biology? The paradox over race is reflected in a scientific community that is fractured by how to deploy race in research. If, as the editors of *Nature Biotechnology* state, 'using genetics to define race is like slicing soup. You can cut wherever you want, but the soup stays mixed',[34] how do we reconcile national efforts to uncover the genetic particularities of racial groups? In creating biobanks that house natural kinds, the colour-line is again drawn, this time underneath the skin, all in the name of science, truth and progress.

Sandra Soo-Jin Lee is a medical anthropologist and Senior Research Scholar at the Stanford Center for Biomedical Ethics at the Stanford University School of Medicine. She researches the social and ethical dimensions of genomic medicine, focusing on race, culture and human genetic variation research, including the implications of pharmacogenomics, racial justice and health disparities, and community-based research ethics.

34 Editorial, *Nature Biotechnology*, vol. 20, no. 7, July 2002, 637.

The rhetoric of race in breast cancer research

KELLY E. HAPPE

ABSTRACT   Since 1998 the *Annual Report to the Nation on the Status of Cancer* has documented the undue burden of breast cancer for women of colour. Geneticists claim that social variables cannot fully explain breast cancer statistics, pointing to evidence that, when black women receive the same health care as Whites, they are still more likely to be diagnosed with aggressive, deadly forms of the disease. Moreover, they claim, racism and traditional risk factors such as reproductive history cannot fully explain why rates are so high among younger black women. The argument that the biology of African-American women—in particular, their genes—explains some percentage of excess incidence and mortality rates presumes that ancestry is a risk factor for breast cancer. It presumes, moreover, that racial categories such as 'African-American', while socially constructed, nevertheless capture the reality of evolutionary history. Indeed, debates about ancestry, race and health disparities demonstrate quite starkly the ways in which 'race' is a rhetorical artefact, reflecting and deflecting the object world of human genetic diversity in ways that shape research agendas and influence public policy debates. Situating the rhetoric of race in genomics research within a larger socio-political context, Happe further argues that the use of race in genomics research is an instantiation of what race theorists Michael Omi and Howard Winant call a 'racial project', defined as 'simultaneously an interpretation, representation, or explanation of racial dynamics, and an effort to reorganize and redistribute resources along particular racial lines'.

S ince 1998 the *Annual Report to the Nation on the Status of Cancer*—a collaboration of the National Cancer Institute, the Centers for Disease Control and Prevention, the American Cancer Society and the North American Association of Central Cancer Registries—has documented the undue burden of breast cancer for women of colour. In 1998 deaths from breast cancer were 28 per cent higher for black women than for white women.[1] In fact, African-American women have the highest breast cancer

1 Lovell A. Jones and Janice A. Chilton, 'Impact of breast cancer on African American women: priority areas for research in the next decade', *American Journal of Public Health*, vol. 92, no. 4, April 2002, 539–42 (540).

mortality rate of any racial or ethnic group in the United States.[2] Moreover, although overall rates for breast cancer are lower than for Whites, rates for breast cancer among young black women are higher and have been so for some time. As epidemiologist Nancy Krieger has observed: 'Combine relatively high incidence and relatively high mortality, and the net result is that US Black women have among the highest breast cancer mortality rates in the world.'[3]

One explanation for this disparity is that environmental risk factors such as diet, reproductive history, environmental racism, lack of access to medical care and unequal treatment by physicians and medical care specialists result in disparities in disease incidence and outcomes. Other researchers, however, claim that social variables cannot fully explain breast cancer statistics, pointing to evidence that, when black women receive the same health care as Whites, they are still more likely to be diagnosed with aggressive, deadly forms of the disease. Moreover, they claim, racism and traditional risk factors such as reproductive history cannot fully explain why rates are so high among younger black women.

Geneticists in particular have shown interest in this statistical anomaly, for breast cancer at a young age is thought to be evidence of inherited susceptibility. For these researchers, the prevalence of genetic mutations may explain why breast cancer is a more dangerous disease for high-risk African-American women and may explain breast cancer cases that other, more well-known risk factors cannot. Geneticists have shown, for example, that women from high-risk African-American families test positive for BRCA1 and BRCA2 mutations. This research is expanding to include the study of the rare population-based 'founder mutations' as well as more common mutations thought to increase risk for breast cancer.

The argument that the biology of African-American women—in particular, their genes—explains some percentage of excess incidence and mortality rates presumes that ancestry is a risk factor for breast cancer. It presumes, moreover, that racial categories such as 'African-American', while socially constructed, nevertheless capture the reality of evolutionary history. Debates about ancestry, race and health disparities demonstrate quite starkly the ways in which 'race' is a rhetorical artefact, reflecting and deflecting the object world of human genetic diversity in ways that shape research agendas and influence public policy debates.[4] Situating the rhetoric of race in

2 Christina A. Clarke, Dee W. West, Brenda K. Edwards, Larry W. Figgs, Jon Kerner and Ann G. Schwartz, 'Existing data on breast cancer in African-American women: what we know and what we need to know', *Cancer*, vol. 97, no. S1 (Supplement), January 2003, 211–21 (211).

3 Nancy Krieger, 'Is breast cancer a disease of affluence, poverty, or both? The case of African American women', *American Journal of Public Health*, vol. 92, no. 4, April 2002, 611–13 (612).

4 Kenneth Burke, *On Symbols and Society*, ed. Joseph R. Gusfield (Chicago: University of Chicago Press 1989).

genomics research within a larger socio-political context, I further argue that the use of race in genomics research is an instantiation of what race theorists Michael Omi and Howard Winant call a 'racial project',

> simultaneously an interpretation, representation, or explanation of racial dynamics, and an effort to reorganize and redistribute resources along particular racial lines. Racial projects connect what race means in a particular discursive practice and the ways in which both social structures and everyday experiences are racially organized, based upon that meaning.[5]

Genomics' attempt to 'reclassify all human illnesses on the basis of detailed molecular characterization', and introduce a 'new molecular taxonomy of illness',[6] often entails using race as a marker for underlying biological difference to explain why some diseases such as cancer, heart disease and hypertension disproportionately impact African Americans. This essay examines one instance of this—the attempt by breast cancer genetics researchers actively to reinterpret differential incidence and mortality. Their interpretation, I maintain, demonstrates how 'race' is a multivalent, yet contested term, organizing our perception of human diversity and imbuing it with meaning that serves different sets of stakeholder interests.

The rhetorical significance of race

The meaning of 'race' has changed quite significantly in the history of biological diversity research. In the seventeenth and eighteenth centuries, scientists devised various classification schemes grounded in the notion that subspecies, or races, of humans existed and could account for observed differences in physical and behavioural traits. The notion of racial inferiority, in turn, was used to justify the brutal practices of European imperialists and, later, by scientists and intellectuals justifying the institution of slavery in revolutionary America.[7]

Beginning with naturalists of the eighteenth century, race has been used primarily to make sense of observed differences in skin colour and other outward physical characteristics, as these were taken to be markers of underlying biological difference among continent-based populations. This

---

5 Michael Omi and Howard Winant, *Racial Formation in the United States: From the 1960s to the 1990s* (London: Routledge 1994), 185.
6 Francis S. Collins, Eric D. Green, Alan E. Guttmacher and Mark S. Guyer, 'A vision for the future of genomics research: a blueprint for the genomic era', *Nature*, vol. 422, 24 April 2003, 835–47 (841).
7 Audrey Smedley, *Race in North America: Origin and Evolution of a Worldview*, 2nd edn (Boulder, CO: Westview Press 1999); Barbara Jeanne Fields, 'Slavery, race and ideology in the United States of America', *New Left Review*, no. 181, May–June 1990, 95–118.

particular notion of 'race' has been the subject of heated debate within various scientific communities, beginning with critiques of early twentieth-century eugenics, prominent attacks in the 1950s and 1960s by anthropologists such as the late Ashley Montagu,[8] Richard Lewontin's 1972 essay demonstrating that most (85 per cent) genetic diversity is found within traditional race groupings rather than between them,[9] and consensus statements by professional societies and the United Nations Educational, Scientific and Cultural Organization (UNESCO) publicly claiming that 'race' is not a legitimate biological concept. When a 'draft' of the human genome was published in 2000, it was accompanied by much fanfare regarding the revelation that humans are, genetically speaking, 99.9 per cent the same.[10]

Humans may differ, on average, by 1 base pair in 1,000 of the 3 billion nucleotides comprising DNA, but the difference matters a great deal in the world of biomedicine. As one observer put it: 'When scientists decoded the human genome, they produced the genetic blueprint for an abstract, generic individual who doesn't really exist.'[11] The appearance and preservation of genetic mutations in geographically and culturally isolated populations interests medical researchers who want to understand both the genetic basis of disease and the relationship between ancestry and risk (e.g. between the sickle cell trait and individuals of African descent). Historically, the concern has been with rare, yet highly penetrant,[12] genetic mutations such as those associated with the so-called Mendelian disorders. The development of sophisticated sequencing technology has enabled researchers to turn their attention to low-penetrant, yet more common alleles that play some role in chronic diseases such as heart disease and cancer. The HapMap project, an international research effort spanning five countries and three years, has produced a map of haplotypes, or sets of single nucleotide polymorphisms (SNPs), thought to be closely linked to functional sections of the genome and thus able to serve as a signpost for the presence of suspected disease alleles. Phase II of the project, documenting over one million SNPs thought common

8   Ashley Montagu (ed.), *The Concept of Race* (New York: Free Press 1964).
9   Richard C. Lewontin, 'The apportionment of human diversity', *Evolutionary Biology*, vol. 6, 1972, 381–98.
10   'Remarks made by the President, Prime Minister Tony Blair of England (via satellite), Dr Francis Collins, Director of the National Human Genome Research Institute, and Dr Craig Venter, President and Chief Scientific Officer, Celera Genomics Corporation, on the completion of the first survey of the entire human genome project', White House press release, 26 June 2000, available at the National Human Genome Research Institute website at http://genome.gov/10001356 (viewed 18 August 2006).
11   Charlie Schmidt, 'Latest HapMap update aims to direct researchers to genetic basis of disease', *Journal of the National Cancer Institute*, vol. 97, no. 22, November 2005, 1638–40 (1638).
12   The word 'penetrance' refers to the proportion of individuals of a particular genotype that expresses its phenotypic effect in a given environment.

to humans, will allow researchers more easily to pursue case control and exploratory studies in order both to determine the degree of risk associated with suspected disease alleles and to locate more regions linked to disease onset.[13]

The development of technology with which to study the complexities of human diversity has not resolved debates about race. It has, in fact, renewed—with much fervour—debates about whether or not patterns of human genetic diversity are homologous to categories of 'race', the latter defined as primary continent of origin.[14] The HapMap Consortium, for instance, while recognizing that no one population would be necessary for inclusion in order to map common SNPs, nevertheless sampled a number of populations that seem to correlate with common understandings of race.[15] The HapMap project is part of the growing debate as to whether or not a genetically inferred primary continent of origin demonstrates a residual reality to socially constructed racial categories: what race critic Jonathan Marks has termed the 'gene pool residual' understanding of race.[16] For many researchers, the answer is 'yes', raising the question of whether the label 'African American' can be a 'proxy' or 'surrogate' for ancestry, a question reaching lay audiences with the publication of biologist Armand Leroi's editorial in the New York Times in March 2005.[17]

Leroi claimed that race is in fact a useful proxy or 'shorthand' for human genetic diversity, criticized the methodology behind Lewontin's 1972 essay as outdated, and cited several articles demonstrating a near correspondence between racial identity and genetic cluster groupings. Cluster analysis, in which researchers divide study subjects into genetically similar subgroupings, can be performed with or without knowledge of individual racial or ethnic identity. That it can be done without knowledge of these identities has

---

13 The International HapMap Consortium, 'A haplotype map of the human genome', *Nature*, vol. 43, October 2005, 1299–320.

14 This definition comes from Neil Risch, Esteban Burchard, Elad Ziv and Hua Tang, 'Categorization of humans in biomedical research: genes, race, and disease', *Genome Biology*, vol. 3, no. 7, July 2002, 1–12. By 'primary' the authors presumably do not mean Africa, although they embrace the 'out of Africa' hypothesis. 'Primary' appears to mean continent reached as a result of 'one or more migration events out of Africa within the last 100,000 years' (3).

15 The populations selected were defined as having 'African, Asian and European ancestry' and included the Yoruba in Nigeria, unrelated Japanese in Tokyo, Han Chinese in Beijing, and thirty samples from Utah.

16 Jonathan Marks, 'The realities of races', 20 April 2005, in *Is Race 'Real'? A Web Forum Organized by the Social Science Research Council*, available on the SSRC website at http://raceandgenomics.ssrc.org/Marks/ (viewed 24 August 2006).

17 Armand Marie Leroi, 'A family tree in every gene', *New York Times*, 14 Mach 2005, A23. For responses, see the forum *Is Race 'Real'? A Web Forum Organized by the Social Science Research Council*, available on the SSRC website at http://raceandgenomics.ssrc.org (viewed 24 August 2006).

led some researchers to conclude that racial identity should never be a part of the geneticist's analysis.[18]

For others, including influential geneticist Neil Risch, it is too soon to jettison the use of racial and ethnic labels. While they share with their critics the goal of individualized, whole-genome analysis, in the short term, they argue, proxies are both technologically and economically necessary.[19] Geneticists further claim that the so-called 'colour-blind' method would impede researchers' attempts to improve minority health since 'results from such studies would be largely derived from the Caucasian majority, with obtained parameter estimates that might not apply to the groups with minority representation'.[20] It further impedes researchers' ability to take into consideration the social dimensions of race and their impact on health outcomes. According to this reasoning, since some studies show a near perfect correspondence between race and genetic cluster groupings, researchers should take into consideration the role of race in disease, both in terms of its social and biological dimensions since

> studies using genetic clusters instead of racial/ethnic labels are likely to simply reproduce racial/ethnic differences, which may or may not be genetic. On the other hand, in the absence of racial/ethnic information, it is tempting to attribute any observed difference between derived genetic clusters to a genetic etiology. Therefore, researchers performing studies without racial/ethnic labels should be wary of characterizing difference between genetically defined clusters as genetic in origin, since social, cultural, economic, behavioral, and other environmental factors may result in extreme confounding.[21]

18 See, for example, James F. Wilson, Michael E. Weale, Alice C. Smith, Fiona Gratix, Benjamin Fletcher, Mark G. Thomas, Neil Bradman and David B. Goldstein, 'Population genetic structure of variable drug response', *Nature Genetics*, vol. 29, no. 3, November 2001, 265–9; 'Genes, drugs, and race' (editorial), *Nature Genetics*, vol. 29, no. 3, November 2001, 239–40; Chiara Romualdi, David Balding, Ivane S. Nasidze, Gregory Risch, Myles Robichaux, Stephen T. Sherry, Mark Stoneking, Mark A. Batzer and Guido Barbujani, 'Patterns of human diversity, within and among continents, inferred from biallelic DNA polymorphisms', *Genome Research*, vol. 12, no. 4, April 2002, 602–12; and Michael Bamshad, Stephen Wooding, Benjamin A. Salisbury and J. Claiborne Stephens, 'Deconstructing the relationship between genetics and race', *Nature Reviews Genetics*, vol. 5, no. 8, August 2004, 598–608.
19 Risch *et al.*, 'Categorization of humans in biomedical research', 2.
20 Ibid., 11.
21 Hua Tang, Tom Quertermous, Beatriz Rodriguez, Sharon L. R. Kardia, Xiaofeng Zhu, Andrew Brown, James S. Pankow, Michael A. Province, Steven C. Hunt, Eric Boerwinkle, Nicholas J. Schork and Neil J. Risch, 'Genetic structure, self-identified race/ethnicity, and confounding in case-control association studies', *American Journal of Human Genetics*, vol. 76, no. 2, February 2005, 268–75 (274).

The race-as-heuristic approach to contemporary diversity studies illus-trates the ways in which 'race' is both scientific concept and rhetorical artefact. As a scientific concept, it organizes and condenses the materiality of the object world: in this case, the materiality of human diversity. As a rhetorical term, it is a partial snapshot of complex patterns of human evolutionary history, rendering certain aspects of human diversity promi-nent (for instance 'primary' continent of origin) and thus meaningful, rendering other aspects of human diversity (such as admixture) insigni-ficant. The rhetorical approach to the study of scientific discourse does not deny the materiality of the object of study; rather, it supposes that the materiality of the object world is accessed—albeit only partially—through the application of scientific theories and the concepts that constitute them. Rhetoric, like the scientific theories it helps to construct, always involves selectivity: literally 'seeing' some objects of study in particular ways while ignoring others, thereby rendering them 'invisible'. As a consequence, scientific rhetoric enables certain questions to be asked and others to be ignored: choices that are an inevitable part of scientific practice.[22] As a perspectival approach to scientific discourse, rhetoric helps us make sense of the influence of what Donna Haraway termed 'situated objectivity', a concept recognizing that we intervene in the material world in ways that reflect certain interests and values.[23]

Discussions about 'race' need not centre on whether or not the term is a faithful representative of reality but should focus rather on *how* it organizes human diversity and, further, what institutional and representational practices enable the production of the concept and overdetermine the meanings with which it operates in scientific practice. 'Linguistic efficacy', biologist Evelyn Fox Keller has argued, depends on the 'technical and natural resources' available to scientists,[24] in this case, technologies for sequencing and mapping the catalogue of human genetic diversity. The acceptability of employing racial categories as rhetorical substitutes for 'population' in turn reflects a 'shared social convention' that permits scientists to talk about the object of study in particular ways.[25] In breast cancer genomics, for example, how is it that the term 'African American' is used to infer ancestry? And when researchers put the term to use, what dominant meanings emerge and become evident? How is ancestry inferred and to what effect?

We must also consider why it *matters* whether or not 'race' or alternative terms such as 'population' are used to represent human diversity. 'Racial and ethnic categories . . . cannot be fully understood outside of the ways in which

22 James J. Bono, 'Science, discourse, and literature: the role/rule of metaphor in science', in Stuart Peterfreund (ed.), *Literature and Science: Theory and Practice* (Boston: Northeastern University Press 1990).

23 Donna Haraway, 'Situated knowledges: the science question in feminism and the privilege of partial perspective', *Feminist Studies*, vol. 14, no. 3, Autumn 1988, 575–99.

24 Evelyn Fox Keller, *Refiguring Life: Metaphors of Twentieth-century Biology* (New York: Columbia University Press 1995), xiii.

25 Ibid., xii.

the process of categorization is materialized in the everyday life of people and the political uses the categories serve.'[26] Indeed, individuals can be grouped any number of ways: depending on the markers used (SNPs, microsatellites etc.), subgroupings will shift accordingly. How we choose to group and, in turn, *name* groups of individuals invariably reflects ideologically inflected habits of mind and are of enormous relevance to the question of whether utilization of the race concept will improve health. While it may be possible to 'find DNA sequences that differ sufficiently between populations to allow correct assignment of major geographical origin with high probability', it is nevertheless also the case that 'genes that are geographically distinctive in their frequencies are not typical of the human genome in general'.[27]

> Race and ancestry are confounded both by genetic heterogeneity within groups and by the widespread mixing of previously isolated populations. The assign-ment of a racial classification to an individual hides the biological information that is needed for intelligent therapeutic and diagnostic decisions. A person classified as 'black' or 'Hispanic' by social convention could have any mixture of ancestries, as defined by continent of origin. Confusing race and ancestry could be potentially devastating for medical practice.[28]

However, if we were to jettison the term 'race' from genetics research, as some have suggested,[29] Hua Tang *et al.* are correct in suggesting that this 'colour-blind' approach would risk hasty conclusions by researchers that differences in disease incidence and outcome are due entirely to genetic factors.[30] However, the long-term goal of individualized genomic medicine presumes the development of methodologies in which non-genetic variables do not exert a confounding effect and that a genomics-inflected explanatory model is appropriate for the study of complex, common diseases. Differential breast cancer rates of incidence and mortality between white and black women is evidence for practitioners in the field of health disparities research that the lived experience of race accounts for observed differences in phenotype.

In what follows, I discuss how, in the field of breast cancer genomics, the meaning of race is variable yet contested, as geneticists and epidemiologists grapple with the complexities of health disparities. While geneticists presume that race is a useful proxy for medically relevant ancestry, the near universal

---

26 Lundy Braun, 'Race, ethnicity, and health: can genetics explain disparities?', *Perspectives in Biology and Medicine*, vol. 45, vol. 2, Spring 2002, 159–74 (168).
27 Marcus W. Feldman, Richard C. Lewontin and Mary-Claire King, 'Race: a genetic melting-pot', *Nature*, vol. 424, July 2003, 374.
28 Ibid.
29 Jacqueline Stevens, 'Racial meaning and scientific methods: changing policies for NIH-sponsored publications reporting human variation', *Journal of Health Politics, Policy and Law*, vol. 28, no. 6, December 2003, 1033–88.
30 Tang *et al.*, 'Genetic structure, self-identified race/ethnicity, and confounding in case-control association studies'.

focus on African ancestry threatens to diminish the practical benefits of biomedicine while reifying notions of essentialized biological difference.

The racialized discourse of breast cancer research

As early as 1996 researchers suggested that breast cancer in black women was, materially speaking, largely a different disease to breast cancer in white women.[31] Evidence of this included statistics showing that black women tended to be diagnosed at an earlier age, with a more advanced stage of the disease and with types of tumours that were difficult to treat.[32] At about the same time the genes BRCA1 and BRCA2 were identified, mutations of which increase risk for breast cancer, some quite significantly so.[33] Since 1996 researchers have been testing African-American women for mutations of these genes.[34] According to at leastone report,[35] the prevalence of BRCA mutations is about the same for high-risk families regardless of African or European ancestry.[36] Genetic screens have further revealed a number of

31 Bruce J. Trock, 'Breast cancer in African American women: epidemiology and tumor biology', *Breast Cancer Research and Treatment*, vol. 40, no. 1, February 1996, 11–24.
32 For example, tumours that were poorly differentiated and difficult to prevent from spreading or were oestrogen-receptor negative and thus resistant to drugs like tamoxifen.
33 Yoshio Miki, Jeff Swensen, Donna Shattuck-Eidens *et al.*, 'A strong candidate for the breast and ovarian cancer susceptibility gene BRCA1', *Science*, vol. 266, 7 October 1994, 66–71; Richard Wooster, Graham Bignell, Jonathan Lancaster *et al.*, 'Identification of the breast cancer susceptibility gene BRCA2', *Nature*, vol. 378, 28 December 1995, 789–92. Inherited breast cancer is thought to explain 5–10 per cent of all breast cancer cases, the majority caused by mutations of BRCA1 and BRCA2 genes.
34 Qing Gao, Gail Tomlinson, Soma Das, Shelly Cummings, Lise Sveen, James Fackenthal, Phil Schumm and Olufunmilayo I. Olopade, 'Prevalence of BRCA1 and BRCA2 mutations among clinic-based African American families with breast cancer', *Human Genetics*, vol. 107, no. 2, August 2000, 186–91; Heather C. Mefford, Lisa Baumbach, Ramesh C. K. Panguluri, Carolyn Whitfield-Broome, Csilla Szabo, Selena Smith, Mary-Claire King, Georgia Dunston, Dominique Stoppa-Lyonnet and Fernando Arena, 'Evidence for a BRCA1 founder mutation in families of West African ancestry', *American Journal of Human Genetics*, vol. 65, no. 2, August 1999, 575–8; Ramesh C. K. Panguluri, Lawrence C. Brody, Rama Modali, Kim Utley, Lucile Adams-Campbell, Agnes A. Day, Carolyn Whitfield-Broome and Georgia M. Dunston, 'BRCA1 mutations in African Americans', *Human Genetics*, vol. 105, nos 1–2, August 1999, 28–31; Tuya Pal, Jenny Permuth-Wey, Tricia Holtje and Rebecca Sutphen, 'BRCA1 and BRCA2 mutations in a study of African American breast cancer patients', *Cancer Epidemiology, Biomarkers and Prevention*, vol. 13, no. 11, November 2004, 1794–9.
35 Olufunmilayo I. Olopade, 'Genetics in clinical cancer care: a promise unfulfilled among minority populations', *Cancer Epidemiology, Biomarkers and Prevention*, vol. 13, no. 11, November 2004, 1683–6.
36 For high-risk women (women with two or more first-degree relatives with breast cancer), the prevalence of BRCA mutations is about 8.7 per cent and above. In the general population, BRCA mutations are thought to be present anywhere from 1 in 300 to 1 in 500 women. See Heidi D. Nelson, Laurie Hoyt Huffman, Rongwei Fu and

mutations never before seen in studies comprised entirely of 'white' subjects.[37]

Founder mutations of the BRCA genes provide additional evidence for researchers that genes may explain health disparities because the identification of founder, or 'ancient', mutations in black women suggests that a different sort of heredity is at work, that of population ancestry, not extended family. Thus, a founder mutation can be detected in two individuals who are geographically or culturally isolated.[38] The 943ins10 mutation of BRCA1, for example, has been detected in women living in the United States, the Bahamas and the Ivory Coast.[39] Although founder mutations have not been identified as frequently among African-American women as they have among other groups, such as women identified as Ashkenazi Jews (it is estimated that the BRCA1 founder mutation 185delAG is found in approximately 3 per cent of persons of Ashkenazi descent),[40] researchers continue to identify potential candidate genes in the hopes that they can explain differential breast cancer rates. (Researchers tend to be interested in founder mutations since they are theoretically much more prevalent in the population than a mutation unique to just one family and thus are of greater public health importance.)

Geneticists have also observed that BRCA breast cancers are biologically similar to breast cancer observed in young black women; they tend to be diagnosed at an early age, and women are typically diagnosed with aggressive, hard-to-treat tumours. These similarities 'suggest that BRCA1 mutations may contribute to breast cancer in a significant proportion of African-American women', although researchers allow that at the moment 'limited data are available from this population to evaluate this possibility'.[41] Nevertheless, the connection between BRCA cancer and cancer in young black women has fuelled interest in the hypothesis that underlying biological difference is a factor. Researchers also believe that common

Emily L. Harris, 'Genetic risk assessment and BRCA mutation testing for breast and ovarian cancer susceptibility: systematic evidence review for the US Preventive Services Task Force', *Annals of Internal Medicine*, vol. 143, no. 5, September 2005, 362–79.

37 Olufunmilayo I. Olopade, James D. Fackenthal, Georgia Dunston, Michael A. Tainsky, Francis Collins and Carolyn Whitfield-Broome, 'Breast cancer genetics in African Americans', *Cancer*, vol. 97, no. S1 (Supplement), January 2003, 236–45.

38 Pal *et al.*, 'BRCA1 and BRCA2 mutations in a study of African American breast cancer patients', 1797.

39 Mefford *et al.*, 'Evidence for a BRCA1 founder mutation in families of West African ancestry'.

40 Jeffery P. Struewing, Dvorah Abeliovich, Tamar Peretz, Naaman Avishai, Michael M. Kaback, Francis S. Collins and Lawrence C. Brody, 'The carrier frequency of the *BRCA1* 185delAG mutation is approximately 1 percent in Ashkenazi Jewish individuals', *Nature Genetics*, vol. 11, October 1995, 198–200.

41 Olopade *et al.*, 'Breast cancer genetics in African Americans', 237.

variations of genes, called polymorphisms, may serve as risk factors for disease in African-American women. These genetic variations do not confer the same amount of risk as the BRCA genes, but nevertheless modify the impact of environmental risk factors and are much more prevalent among populations.[42] Of significance are polymorphisms of genes that may impact metabolism of oestrogen and environmental contaminants.[43]

Patterns of genetic variation, of which BRCA mutations, BRCA founder mutations and polymorphisms are evidence, suggest the importance of evaluating ancestry in order to understand breast cancer disparities. The 'unique spectrum' of observed BRCA mutations, for example, suggests that, while there is substantial variation within groups of women identified as 'African American', this variation is distinct from patterns observed in other racial and ethnic groups: what Risch *et al.* claim is the difference between variation and differentiation; in their exact words, the 'greatest genetic structure that exists in the human population occurs at the racial level', 'race' being broadly defined as primary continent of origin.[44] Data from genetics studies are used by researchers to categorize African-American women into a single, biologically delimited population.

This classificatory move is only possible, however, if one assumes that health outcomes are principally influenced by an inferred 'African' ancestry, an assumption made evident by researchers' choice to draw parallels between breast cancer statistics in the United States and Africa. Some patterns of the disease are suggestive of shared ancestry: when adjusted for age, young women in some African nations exhibit a higher rate for breast cancer, much like young black women in the United States. One study concluded: 'The parallels between African-American and sub-Saharan African breast cancer suggests the possible effects of hereditary factors, and these influences may cause the younger age distribution that is seen among these patient populations to persist.'[45] Another study suggested: 'It is likely that the shared genetic

---

42 Because BRCA mutations are rare and explain only 5–10 per cent of breast cancer cases, researchers are showing increased interest in common polymorphisms that increase risk for breast cancer, including polymorphisms that are more prevalent among 'racial' groups.

43 Chantal Guillemette, Robert C. Millikan, Beth Newman and David E. Housman, 'Genetic polymorphisms in uridine diphospho-glucuronosyltransferase 1A1 and association with breast cancer among African Americans', *Cancer Research*, vol. 60, no. 4, February 2000, 950–6; Francine Laden, Naoko Ishibe, Susan E. Hankinson, Mary S. Wolff, Dorota M. Gertig, David J. Hunter and Karl T. Kelsey, 'Polychlorinated biphenyls, cytochrome P450 1A1, and breast cancer risk in the Nurses' Health Study', *Cancer Epidemiology, Biomarkers and Prevention*, vol. 11, no. 12, December 2002, 1560–5.

44 Risch *et al.*, 'Categorization of humans in biomedical research: genes, race, and disease', 4.

45 Alero Fregene and Lisa A. Newman, 'Breast cancer in sub-Saharan Africa: how does it relate to breast cancer in African-American women?', *Cancer*, vol. 103, no. 8, April 2005, 1540–50 (1548).

background of Africans and U.S. African Americans contributes to the greater susceptibility to early-onset breast cancer in both groups but this has not been evaluated carefully.'[46] These statements suggest a tendency on the part of researchers to privilege the African ancestry of admixed populations. Although many of the same researchers acknowledge the very real fact of genetic admixture, they nevertheless consider African ancestry to be the only relevant variable in assessing breast cancer risk.[47] Genetic variations that increase risk for breast cancer are racially marked in references to 'shared genetic background'; African ancestry stands in, metonymically, for complex and diverse heredity.

Yet race is a poor marker of genetic lineage as 'by some estimates more than three quarters of Americans who identify themselves as black or African American have a blood relative who identifies themselves as white or Caucasian'.[48] Indeed, the literature on founder mutations often ignores the very real possibility that the 'African' founder mutation 943ins10 could be detected in 'white' women. The fact that founder mutations are rarely found in black study subjects also suggests that they will not be detected in the vast majority of African-American women. In one data set published in 2003 over sixty BRCA1 mutations had been detected in African-American and African families *as well as* families with no reported African ancestry. One of these mutations is the 943ins10 founder mutation of the BRCA1 gene.[49]

In a case of intractable dominant paradigms in the practice of scientific research, not dissimilar to the cases Thomas Kuhn documented,[50] researchers tend to overlook these anomalies and routinely refer to 'unique' mutations never previously reported as evidence that African-American women are biologically distinct, presumably understood to be a race unto themselves: 'Despite the substantial heterogeneity of ethnic ancestry that exists within many African-American families', wrote one research group, 'a disproportionate risk for breast cancer mortality has been consistently demonstrated for women who identify themselves as African American'.[51] If human evolutionary patterns permitted the construction of such neatly circumscribed populations of persons, one would expect other breast cancer patients to be similarly partitioned. However, although novel mutations are

46 Olopade *et al.*, 'Breast cancer genetics in African Americans', 241. Olopade *et al.* chalk this up to a lack of interest in the role of genetic variants in black breast cancer patients and conclude by calling for more research.

47 Ibid., 242.

48 Otis W. Brawley, 'Population categorization and cancer statistics', *Cancer and Metastasis Reviews*, vol. 22, no. 1, March 2003, 11–19 (14).

49 Olopade *et al.*, 'Breast cancer genetics in African Americans', 238, 240.

50 Thomas S. Kuhn, *The Structure of Scientific Revolutions* [1962] (Chicago: University of Chicago Press 1970).

51 Fregene and Newman, 'Breast cancer in sub-Saharan Africa: how does it relate to breast cancer in African-American women?', 1540–1.

nothing unusual in white subjects (many of the reported mutations of BRCA1 and BRCA2 appear in just one family), researchers never talk about white women as biologically distinct from other races, and for whom genetic mutations can explain higher rates of incidence, lower mortality and histologically distinct tumours. The *de facto*—and correct—assumption is that white women are not a 'race', but a biologically diverse population with multiple ancestral lines that all play a role in breast cancer risk. That African-American women are classified in this fashion suggests that race represents the epistemological commitments of researchers as much as it does the truth of African ancestry and its medical relevance.

Racializing breast cancer susceptibility is not without potentially serious consequences for the health care of black women. Here the case of sickle cell anaemia and sickle cell trait is instructive.

> If sickle-cell disease is suspected, then the correct diagnostic approach is not simply to determine the patient's race, but to ask whether they have African, Mediterranean or South Indian ancestry. To use genotype effectively in making diagnostic and therapeutic decisions, it is not race that is relevant, but both intra- and trans-continental contributions to a person's ancestry.[52]

To be sure:

> Sickle-cell anemia is not a 'race specific' disease that reflects the underlying genetic make-up of West Africans and African Americans. The higher prevalence of sickle-cell disease in African Americans is in a very important sense an artifact of classification. In Brazil, for example, where many African Americans would be considered white the prevalence of a disease such as sickle cell might be very similar between people considered white. By virtue of ancestry, not all African Americans are at risk of sickle-cell disease, whereas some white populations and Latinos have a risk which is not well documented.[53]

If inherited susceptibility to breast cancer results from the confluence of multiple ancestries, it would be unwise to racialize women identified as African American by targeting them for genetic screens and by privileging African ancestry over others when assessing genetic risk. Until the long-term promise of individually tailored risk assessment and treatment is realized, it is most likely the case that 'the false universalization of heritable traits poses fewer health risks than a false particularization of such traits'.[54]

---

52 Feldman, Lewontin and King, 'Race: a genetic melting-pot'.
53 Braun, 'Race, ethnicity, and health', 167.
54 Jacqueline Stevens, 'Eve is from Adam's rib, the earth is flat, and race comes from genes', 30 June 2005, in *Is Race 'Real'? A Web Forum Organized by the Social Science Research Council*, available on the SSRC website at http://raceandgenomics.ssrc.org/ Stevens/ (viewed 1 September 2006).

All of this presumes, however, the explanatory power of genomics research with regard to understanding, and eventually eliminating, health disparities. As social epidemiologist Nancy Krieger has observed: 'The interpretations we offer of observed average differences in health status across socially-delimited groups reflects our theoretical frameworks, not ineluctable facts of nature.'[55] Geneticists are reinterpreting breast cancer statistics as evidence of inherited susceptibility, especially with regard to elevated rates among young black women.

As already stated, breast cancer mortality rates among black women in the United States are unparalleled and show evidence of a disturbing pattern. Between 1973 and 1990 incidence in black women under fifty increased by over 16 per cent while the increase for white women in this same age-group increased by 6 per cent.[56] Between 1969 and 1997 the age-adjusted death rate for white women dropped 15 per cent while it increased by 22 per cent for African-American women.[57] Rates are very high among older black women. Crude rates of breast cancer in women younger than fifty years of age between 1992 and 1997 were actually lower for black than for white women, although when adjusted for age they were slightly higher. 'In addition, regardless of race or age adjustment, rates of breast cancer for women < 50 years are one-eighth to one-tenth the rates for women age > 50 years, underscoring the low absolute risk of breast cancer in women age < 50 years compared with older women.'[58] One interpretation of these historical shifts is the following:

> Beyond the clinical trials, epidemiologic assessment of the US population suggests biologic/genetic differences may have been overemphasized. Often unappreciated is the fact that black–white mortality was very similar in the 1970s and the disparity in mortality rate has grown every year from 1981 onward.[59]

Yet 'biologic' differences are precisely what geneticists want to emphasize. The biological difference theory is grounded in the argument by researchers that social variables cannot explain observed health disparities. According to this reasoning, when black women have the same access to health care and are diagnosed at the same stage of breast cancer, they are still more likely to die from the disease in part because they are diagnosed with histologically distinct tumours. The fact that African-American women

55 Nancy Krieger, 'If "race" is the answer, what is the question?—on "race," racism, and health: an epidemiologist's perspective', 20 April 2005, in *Is Race 'Real'? A Web Forum Organized by the Social Science Research Council*, available on the SSRC website at http://raceandgenomics.ssrc.org/Krieger/ (viewed 1 September 2006).
56 Trock, 'Breast cancer in African American women', 12.
57 Clarke *et al.*, 'Existing data on breast cancer in African-American women', 211.
58 Ibid., 218–19.
59 Otis W. Brawley, 'Cancer and health disparities', *Cancer and Metastasis Reviews*, vol. 22, no. 1, March 2003, 7–9 (8).

maintain a survival deficit compared to white women, even after controlling for stage of disease at diagnosis and other factors associated with socioeconomic status such as treatment and obesity, suggests the possibility of biological differences associated with race.[60]

The biological/genetic argument rests on the assumption that social variables cannot entirely explain observed differences in health disparities, although few if any studies are referenced as evidence. Researchers hastily conclude that an inherent, hereditary and recalcitrant biological reality of race is the only possible explanation for observed differences when all other risk factors and social variables are controlled for, reasoning not at all dissimilar to that which informed the claims of the authors of *The Bell Curve* in the mid-1990s.[61]

> The statement most often made in the conclusions of such investigations is that the black–white difference *persists after adjustment for SES* [socio-economic status], and that this indicates another source of susceptibility, frequently ascribed to 'genetic' factors. This conclusion is based on the mistaken belief that the groups have been made exchangeable with respect to socially related exposures.[62]

There are many reasons why racial groups are not interchangeable when measuring variables such as socio-economic status, including the differential impact of education (similar levels of education do not necessarily result in similar incomes and employment opportunities) and a dissimilar experience of income (for example debt-to-income ratio may mean that income carries less beneficial impact for black Americans), leading one group of epidemiologists to conclude that 'adjusting at the individual level for an effect that occurs causally at the society level cannot logically produce a meaningful model of disease etiology, no matter how refined the measures'.[63]

The problem of 'residual confounding' is a significant one, overlooked in the pursuit of genetic explanations for cancer disparities between black and white women, reflecting perhaps 'the influence of social ideology on the conduct of medical science'.[64] Residual confounding may well play a role in breast cancer studies. When one adjusts for stage of disease and access to health care, factors such as race and class can nevertheless serve as variables that can explain the kinds of breast tumours diagnosed in black women:

60 Trock, 'Breast cancer in African American women', 18.
61 Richard Herrnstein and Charles Murray, *The Bell Curve: Intelligence and Class Structure in American Life* (New York: Simon and Schuster 1996).
62 Jay S. Kaufman, Richard S. Cooper and Daniel L. McGee, 'Socioeconomic status and health in Blacks and Whites: the problem of residual confounding and the resiliency of race', *Epidemiology*, vol. 8, no. 6, October 1997, 621–8 (622) (emphasis in the original).
63 Ibid., 627.
64 Ibid.

Race is a social variable, not an inherent biologic variable. It is clear that, compared with white women, a disproportionately higher proportion of black women present with later-stage disease and that, within any one stage, a higher proportion of blacks than whites have poor prognostic markers, such as higher pathologic grade and estrogen receptor-negative disease. Gordon and colleagues have shown that low education level and low income are associated with the diagnosis of estrogen receptor-negative tumors, which suggests that factors associated with socio-economic status may influence the biologic behavior of breast cancer.[65]

Not only is it difficult to control for all socio-cultural factors that can contribute to disease risk, this quotation from cancer researcher Otis Brawley supports the argument that, even when researchers are reasonably confident that they have, class and race operate as confounding variables in ways that they sometimes ignore or simply do not understand.

Geneticists are most eager to address the issue of elevated breast cancer rates among young African-American women, since young age of onset suggests inherited susceptibility. According to the two-hit hypothesis, some women are born with a deleterious mutation of a breast cancer susceptibility gene (one 'hit') and are thus more vulnerable (and at an earlier age) since a second hit is quite likely due to the vagaries of cellular replication and women's exposure to environmental mutagens. Statistics showing that, when adjusted for age, young black women are at greater risk for breast cancer than their white counterparts suggest for geneticists that race-based inherited susceptibility is a factor. That common risk factors such as reproductive history do not explain these higher-than-expected rates appears to add some credibility to the heredity thesis. Epidemiologists have shown, for example, that, when fertility rates are higher for black study subjects, breast cancer rates are also higher, defying the so-called 'hormonal hypothesis'. According to Nancy Krieger:

> in contrast to the hormonal hypothesis' prediction regarding higher white breast cancer rates, among women under age 40, commencing with the Third National Cancer Survey, the incidence of breast cancer among black women has exceeded and risen more quickly than that of whites, and in 1980 was 30% higher.[66]

---

65 Otis W. Brawley, 'Disaggregating the effects of race and poverty on breast cancer outcomes', *Journal of the National Cancer Institute*, vol. 94, no. 7, April 2002, 471–3 (471).

66 Nancy Krieger, 'Exposure, susceptibility, and breast cancer risk: a hypothesis regarding exogenous carcinogens, breast tissue development, and social gradients, including black/white differences, in breast cancer incidence', *Breast Cancer Research and Treatment*, vol. 13, no. 3, October 1989, 205–23 (207). Since the publication of Krieger's article, fertility rates among African-American women have fallen and are near those of Whites. See Jane Dawler Dye, *Fertility of American Women: June 2004*, Report P20-555 (Washington, D.C.: US Census Bureau 2005), available on the US Census Bureau website at www.census.gov/prod/2005pubs/p20-555.pdf (viewed 15 September 2006).

For Krieger and others, one possible explanation for this statistical anomaly is that black women are more likely to be exposed to a certain class of chemicals known as organochlorines, or OCCs, that increase breast cancer risk. The theory is that organochlorines, such as the pesticide DDT and the class of chemicals known as PCBs, are 'oestrogenic' and thus increase breast cancer risk.[67] Some studies have documented a link between OCC exposure and breast cancer risk,[68] while others have not.[69] When race is taken into account, some studies suggest a connection between OCC exposure and breast cancer

67 The chemicals in question are ubiquitous in the environment and, in the bodies of wildlife and humans, do not break down easily and tend to 'bioaccumulate', that is, the amount of synthetic chemical body burden is much higher at the top of the food chain than at the bottom. This explains why concentrations are high in fish and particularly high in humans who depend on fish for food. Synthetic chemicals that are classified as 'persistent' (and thus likely to bioaccumulate) have been termed 'POPs', or 'persistent organic pollutants'. The UN has listed twelve POPs of greatest concern to scientists and environmental health activists. See Michelle Allsopp, Ruth Stringer and Paul Johnston, *Unseen Poisons: Levels of Organochlorine Chemicals in Human Tissues*, Greenpeace Research Laboratories Technical Report (Amsterdam: Greenpeace International 1998), available online at http://archive.greenpeace.org/toxics/reports/unseenpo.pdf (viewed 1 September 2006). And, as Sandra Steingraber notes in her recent book, *Having Faith: An Ecologist's Journey to Motherhood* (Cambridge, MA: Perseus Publishing 2001), although breast-fed infants are not included in the typical 'chart' of the food chain, it is important to note that they occupy its highest slot since human milk is a repository for human food intake. Many synthetic chemicals bioaccumulate in human breast milk making it one of the most contaminated foods on the planet. See Steingraber, *Having Faith*, and Allsopp, Stringer and Johnston, *Unseen Poisons*. Richard Jackson, director of the National Center for Environmental Health at the Centers for Disease Control has claimed: 'If you compared the legally allowable levels of toxic chemicals in cow's milk with levels of toxic chemicals in human milk, you would conclude that half the human milk in the United States would be unfit for sale under FDA guidelines.' Richard Jackson, 'Unburdening ourselves', *Silent Spring Review*, Fall 2000, 6–7, available at the Silent Spring Institute website at http://library.silentspring.org/publications/pdfs/ssi_revfall00.pdf (viewed 1 September 2006).
68 Mary S. Wolff, Paolo G. Toniolo, Eric W. Lee, Marilyn Rivera and Neil Dubin, 'Blood levels of organochlorine residues and risk of breast cancer', *Journal of the National Cancer Institute*, vol. 85, no. 8, April 1993, 648–52; Éric Dewailly, Pierre Ayotte and Sylvie Dodin, 'Could the rising levels of estrogen receptor in breast cancer be due to estrogenic pollutants?', *Journal of the National Cancer Institute*, vol. 89, no. 12, June 1997, 888–9; Éric Dewailly, Sylvie Dodin, René Verreault, Pierre Ayotte, Louise Sauvé, Jacques Morin and Jacques Brisson, 'High organochlorine body burden in women with estrogen receptor-positive breast cancer', *Journal of the National Cancer Institute*, vol. 86, no. 3, February 1994, 232–4.
69 David J. Hunter, Susan E. Hankinson, Francine Laden, Graham A. Colditz, JoAnn E. Manson, Walter C. Willett, Frank Speizer and Mary S. Wolff, 'Plasma organochlorine levels and the risk of breast cancer', *New England Journal of Medicine*, vol. 337, no. 18, October 1997, 1253–8; Steven D. Stellman, Mirjana V. Djordjevic, Julie A. Britton, Joshua E. Muscat, Marc L. Citron, Margaret Kemeny, Erna Busch and Lin Gong, 'Breast cancer risk in relation to adipose concentrations of organochlorine pesticides and polychlorinated biphenyls in Long Island, New York', *Cancer Epidemiology, Biomarkers and Prevention*, vol. 9, no. 11, November 2000, 1241–9.

risk among black women, although the statistical significance of this association is somewhat weak.[70] What these studies have consistently shown is that, when race is taken into account, the body burden of carcinogens is greater for black women than for white women, sometimes quite significantly so.[71] In one study, researchers observed that levels of DDE (the principal metabolite of DDT) and PCBs were higher in African-American than in white women.[72] African-American women with breast cancer also had higher DDE and PCB levels than their white counterparts. Indeed, 'studies over the past 30 years consistently have found OC compounds to be present at higher levels in African-Americans compared to whites, and this pattern appears to continue'.[73]

Exposure to dangerous chemicals may explain higher rates among young African-American women, since developing breasts are more vulnerable to environmental toxins.[74] 'Together, these findings imply that breast cancer in women occurs as a generalized response to systemic carcinogens operating within the breasts' most active tissue.'[75] An alternative framework would examine the dynamic interplay of race—socially conceived—and biology.

> Instead of a single-minded focus on identifying race- or ethnic-specific polymorphisms, or on studying cultural behaviors which fail to acknowledge the diversity and changing character of culture, an alternative framework of analysis would examine the potential biological mechanisms through which life experience can affect health. Such an analysis would explore the dynamic nature of the

70 Mary S. Wolff, Julie A. Britton and Valerie P. Wilson, 'Environmental risk factors for breast cancer among African-American women', *Cancer*, vol. 97, no. S1 (Supplement), January 2003, 289–310.
71 The racial stratification of chemical exposures is well documented. In one 1977 study, levels of DDT were twice that of white subjects and researchers were twice as likely to find traces of lindane in black tissue samples. F. W. Kutz, A. R. Yobs and S. C. Strassman, 'Racial stratification of organochlorine insecticide residue in human adipose tissue', *Journal of Occupational Medicine*, vol. 9, 19 September 1977, 619–22.
72 Robert Millikan, Emily DeVoto, Eric J. Duell, Chiu-Kit Tse, David A. Savitz, James Beach, Sharon Edmiston, Susan Jackson and Beth Newman, 'Dichlorodiphenyldichloroethene, polychlorinated biphenyls, and breast cancer among African-American and white women in North Carolina', *Cancer Epidemiology, Biomarkers and Prevention*, vol. 9, no. 11, November 2000, 1233–40.
73 Wolff, Britton and Wilson, 'Environmental risk factors for breast cancer among African-American women', 294.
74 H. McGregor, C. E. Land, K. Choi, S. Tokuoka, P. I. Liu, T. Wakabayashi and G. W. Beebe, 'Breast cancer incidence among atomic bomb survivors, Hiroshima and Nagasaki 1950–69', *Journal of the National Cancer Institute*, vol. 59, no. 3, September 1977, 799–811; Jose Russo, Lee K. Tay and Irma H. Russo, 'Differentiation of the mammary gland and susceptibility to carcinogenesis', *Breast Cancer Research and Treatment*, vol. 2, no. 1, March 1982, 5–73; Trock, 'Breast cancer in African American women'; Wolff, Britton and Wilson, 'Environmental risk factors for breast cancer among African-American women'.
75 Krieger, 'Exposure, susceptibility, and breast cancer risk', 210.

relationship between humans and their social and physical environment and the effects of this interaction on the expression of genes, rather than ascribing an exaggerated biological meaning to a string of nucleotides. Such an analysis has the potential to provide explanations for differences in prevalence of disease or disease-related mortality, as well as puzzling features of the natural history of disease, such as the earlier age of onset of breast cancer in African Americans. In other words, causal explanations of disease would look at the disease experience of individuals or socially constructed population categories in the context of, not separate from, the social and physical environment.[76]

Conclusion and implications

For hundreds of years, scientists have devised methods of visually and conceptually organizing human groups. The concept 'race' has been one such way of ordering biological diversity into methodologically convenient types not only to facilitate the testing of scientific hypotheses but also, as the history of scientific racism demonstrates, to provide powerful arguments for white superiority.

Like all classification schemata, however, that based on the assumption of human races is arbitrary, albeit strategic and self-serving. Over time, the techniques for measuring race failed to provide cogent evidence and this failure necessitated the adoption of new classification tools based on the notion of 'population'. In theory, the development of sophisticated tools of genetic analysis enables scientists to construct complex narratives of human evolution and migration. In practice, what emerges in breast cancer research is a narrative of human diversity in which the ancestry of African-American women is described along the lines of conventional and supposedly legitimate notions of biological race. Not only do scientists routinely and explicitly use the word 'race' in referring to their study subjects, their research questions seem designed to prove what they already believe, namely, that black women are members of a racial, not a population, group. Researchers are in effect confusing genetic diversity with racial diversity: finding a unique spectrum of genetic variables in black study subjects is biological evidence of the history of human migration not of racial types.

The racialism in breast cancer research casts serious doubt on its scientific legitimacy. By privileging African ancestry, the importance of other, equally important, genetic variables are overlooked by researchers. Socially defined race may be an appropriate category for epidemiologists and medical sociologists, but it is decidedly inappropriate if the research questions entail searching for biological markers of group membership and the demarcation of at-risk populations. As public health researcher Larry Figgs put it, the racial categories typically employed by researchers

76 Braun, 'Race, ethnicity, and health', 168–9.

infer minimal information about biology or genetics—information that is fundamentally important to contemporary cancer models. Second, although they are convenient, these categories do not represent distinct boundaries, and their meanings overlap with other terms. Finally, allowing respondents to use 'fluid' identity criteria decreases statistical resolution by increasing the likelihood of misclassification.[77]

Some critics have called for geneticists to stop using the term 'race' altogether and to refrain from any suggestion that advances in genomics can improve the health of minority groups.[78] Jettisoning the language of race in genomics is an idea worth taking seriously, not only in the interest of advancing the methodologies of health disparities research, but in raising public awareness of issues of poverty, discrimination and the dismantling of our public health infrastructure. The genetics framework not only privileges African ancestry; it privileges heredity writ large in its explanation of disease. African-American women are being classified as at-risk not because of their shared experiences of poverty and environmental racism but because of shared biology, whether in the form of rare mutations or more common variations of susceptibility genes. As a 'racial project', breast cancer genomics represents race in a way that reshapes our perception of the lived experience of African-American women and shifts the burden of proof in explaining disease to geneticists, not policymakers: a shift that impacts not just women of colour but all women at risk for breast cancer.

Kelly E. Happe is an assistant professor of rhetorical studies in the Department of Communication at Northern Illinois University. Her articles on genetics have appeared in *Rhetoric and Public Affairs*, *Journal of Medical Humanities* and *GeneWatch*, the magazine of the Council for Responsible Genetics, and another is forthcoming in *New Genetics and Society*. This essay is part of a larger project that examines the rhetoric of race, gender and risk in scientific discourses about ovarian and breast cancer.

77 Larry W. Figgs, 'Breast cancer research among African-American women: accurate racial categories?', *Cancer*, vol. 97, no. S1 (Supplement), January 2003, 335–41 (338).
78 Stevens, 'Racial meaning and scientific methods'.

Against racial medicine

JOSEPH L. GRAVES, Jr AND MICHAEL R. ROSE

ABSTRACT   Some scholars claim that recent studies of human genetic variation validate the existence of human biological races and falsify the idea that human races are socially constructed misconceptions. They assert that analyses of DNA polymorphisms unambiguously partition individuals into groups that are very similar to lay conceptions of race. Furthermore, they propose that this partitioning allows us to identify specific loci that can explain contemporary health disparities between the supposed human races. From this, it appears that racial medicine has risen again. In this essay Graves and Rose construct a case against racial medicine. Biological races in other species are strongly differentiated genetically. Because human populations do not have such strong genetic differentiation, they are not biological races. Nonetheless, the lack of population genetic knowledge among biomedical researchers has led to spuriously racialized human studies. But human populations are not genetically disjoint. Social dominance may lead to medical differences between socially constructed races. In order to resolve these issues, medicine should take both social environment and population genetics into account, instead of dubious 'races' that inappropriately conflate the two.

Racial medicine has risen again

Charles B. Davenport, one of the most respected scientists of the first decades of the twentieth century, argued that laziness was a hereditary trait. Davenport claimed in particular that laziness was a heredity character of Southern Whites. Later epidemiological studies determined that 'white trash' laziness was actually the result of heavy infections caused by the nematode necator americanus.[1] But, for Davenport and many other biologists of his time, the phenotypic differences displayed by particular populations were proof positive of the existence of human races. They believed that these races differed in readily observable features, such as skin colour and body proportions, and also in those they could not directly observe, such as intellect, morality, character, disease predisposition and

---

1 Charles B. Davenport, 'The hereditary factor in pellagra' (1917), quoted in Allan Chase, *The Legacy of Malthus: The Social Costs of the New Scientific Racism* (New York: Alfred A. Knopf 1977), 203.

resistance. In 1921, for example, Ernest Zimmerman published a report on differences in the manifestation of syphilis in Blacks and Whites. Such thinking helped to sanction the now infamous Tuskegee syphilis experiment.[2] Modern biologists recoil with horror when asked to revisit this sad episode in the history of science.

The rationale for the Tuskegee experiment was the underlying assumption that the Negro was genetically inferior to Whites. Thus, the perceived differences in incidence rates and progression of disease were thought to reside in characteristics intrinsic to the race, as opposed to the social conditions under which visibly darker-skinned persons of African descent lived in the United States. (It is significant that many 'white Americans' have African ancestors but 'pass as white', an anomaly to which we will return below.) Therefore, the Tuskegee experiment suffered not only from its moral shortcomings, but also from poor experimental design. The results of the experiment could not have distinguished between any genetically based difference in disease progression, since many environmental and social differences between African Americans and the Swedish cohorts with which they were to be compared were not properly controlled. With hindsight, the scientific problems of this experiment are obvious. What is not recognized is that modern discussions of race and medicine have not moved very far beyond the misconceptions that gave birth to the Tuskegee research programme.

In 2001 the *New England Journal of Medicine* featured an exchange between two physicians, Robert Schwartz and Alistair Wood. Schwartz argued that racial profiling in medical research was unsound because biological races did not exist in the human species, citing the 1999 statement of the American Anthropological Association. Wood attempted to rebut Schwartz. He pointed out that human populations have different frequencies of genes. For example, he argued that both black Americans and Africans have a high frequency of a cytochrome P allele (CYP2D6) that encodes low activity for that enzyme. Furthermore, this allele is virtually absent in European and Asian populations. Knowing whether groups differ in this enzyme is important because it affects the metabolic effects of several drugs. Wood continued with several examples of this kind, yet he never explained how biological races were defined, whether those definitions applied to our species or, finally, whether the groups he described in his essay fit conventional biological definitions of 'race'.[3]

Likewise, in 2002, Sally Satel, a fellow of the American Enterprise Institute, wrote, citing essentially the same arguments as Wood, that she used racial

---

2 James H. Jones, *Bad Blood: The Tuskegee Syphilis Experiment* (New York: The Free Press and London: Collier Macmillan 1981), 28.

3 Robert S. Schwartz, 'Racial profiling in medical research', and Alistair J. J. Wood, 'Racial differences in responses to drugs—pointers to genetic differences', *New England Journal of Medicine*, vol. 344. no. 18, May 2001, 1392–3 and 1393–6, respectively.

profiling in her medical practice.[4] A year ago, the *New York Times* published an op-ed piece entitled 'A Family Tree in Every Gene' by Armand Leroi of Imperial College, London. In this article, Leroi suggested that recent genetic research supported the idea of human racial differentiation because it was relatively easy to classify humans into distinct groups if enough genetic markers were used.[5] Given these recent claims, it appears that the way has been cleared for a return to Davenport's emphasis on the genetic origins of racial disparities in susceptibility to disease: a return to racial medicine.

The identification of human races is not based on cogent biology

While humans have always recognized the existence of physical differences between groups, they haven't always described those differences in racial terms. Racial theories of human differentiation were not a consistent theme of the ancient world, and really did not begin to flourish until after the European voyages of discovery in the fifteenth century. European naturalists of the eighteenth century were divided about the characterization of human differences. Almost all agreed that there was only one human species, yet they disagreed about whether there was a legitimate way to rank the various groups of humans hierarchically. For example, Carl Linneaus's *Systema Naturae* (1735) classified human races partly on the basis of subjectively determined behavioural traits. It is not clear, however, what Linnaeus meant by the use of the term 'race'. It seems that his classification scheme was describing subspecies of humans based on morphological features. According to it, European traits were clearly superior to others, and Africans were assigned the lowest rung in the hierarchy.

Such racist ideas were transplanted to America during colonial times, along with other biological absurdities. During American chattel slavery, the socially defined race of the offspring of slavemasters and slave women was 'Negro'. Virginia law classified Eston Hemmings, who was 87.5 per cent European according to genetic ancestry, as 'Negro'. Geneticists now suspect that Thomas Jefferson was his father, based on family genealogies and a genetic marker specific to the Jefferson family found in Eston's descendants.

The one-drop rule (also called 'hypo-descent') in the United States differs from definitions of 'blackness' in Canada, Mexico, Britain and Brazil. Individuals, therefore, could move from one country to another and be classified differently according to the social custom. Indeed, in the United States, individuals have been born as a member of one race and died as a

4 Sally Satel, 'I am a racially profiling doctor', *New York Times Sunday Magazine*, 5 May 2002.

5 Armand Marie Leroi, 'A family tree in every gene', *New York Times*, 14 Mach 2005, A23; A. W. F. Edwards, 'Human genetic diversity: Lewontin's fallacy', *Bioessays*, vol. 25, no. 8, August 2003, 798–801.

member of another. European ethnic groups, such as the Irish and Italians, did not become 'white' until the twentieth century. Such 'races' are clearly based on social conventions, as opposed to biological measures of genetic ancestry. Socially produced racial ideology from the very beginning influenced the collection and interpretation of data relating to human biological variation.

Ashley Montagu was one of the first scholars to analyse the idea of race in humans explicitly as a social construction. Montagu pointed out that human physical variation was discordant.[6] For example, sub-Saharan Africans, East Indians and Australian aborigines have dark skin but differ in other anatomical traits, such as bodily proportions, skull proportions, hair type and ear wax consistency. More recently, C. Loring Brace has shown that, while physical features can be used to demonstrate the likely geographical origin of an individual skeleton, these features do not allow the unambiguous classification of races.[7] Geneticist Sewall Wright made the same point concerning discordance in his discussion of the genetic differentiation of the races of mankind.[8]

Human populations are not biological races

The measurement and apportionment of human diversity have been core issues in genetic research. This work has focused on the question of whether human genetic variation has a significant substructure.[9] Sewall Wright developed hierarchical population statistics in order to partition genetic variation within a species. Wright's statistics treat variation at the level of breeding populations (demes) within regions (DR), regions within primary subdivisions (RS), and primary subdivisions within the total species (ST). Wright argued that the last statistic was the best measure of subspecies differentiation, 'subspecies' being the term used by taxonomists as an equivalent for biological race. Such population subdivision can be calculated at individual genetic loci or at numerous genetic loci simultaneously. Wright's subspecies statistic (referred to formally as F_{st}) can range between 0 and 1.0, a value of 0 (zero) indicating complete lack of genetic differentiation between major groups. He suggested that the minimal threshold for the existence of racial differentiation would be an

6 Ashley Montagu, *Man's Most Dangerous Myth: The Fallacy of Race*, rev. 5th edn (New York: Oxford University Press 1974).
7 C. Loring Brace, 'Region does not mean "race"—reality versus convention in forensic anthropology', *Journal of Forensic Sciences*, vol. 40, no. 2, March 1995, 29–33.
8 Sewall Wright, *Evolution and the Genetics of Populations. Vol. 4: Variability within and among Natural Populations* (Chicago: University Chicago Press 1978).
9 Robert H. Podolsky and Timothy P. Holtsford, 'Population structure of morphological traits in *Clarkia dudleyana*: I. Comparison of F_{st} between allozymes and morphological traits', *Genetics*, vol. 140, no. 2, June 1995, 733–44.

F_{st} of 0.25 or more, with moderate variation between populations arising with F_{st} values between 0.15 and 0.25. He examined individual loci from a variety of species, finding a range of differentiation of about 0.02 to 0.50. Using six human blood group loci, he estimated that F_{st} averaged about 0.12 between the human races. This F_{st} value did not come close to 0.25, Wright's pre-established threshold for the existence of subspecies, though human populations within geographic regions share more alleles with each other than they do with populations from other regions.

Subsequent studies of human genetic variation, including whole genome analyses, have generally also found estimates of F_{st} to be much less than Wright's critical value. Genetic substructure does exist in humans, but there are no natural divisions in our species equivalent to biological races. Recently, Jeffrey Long and Rick Kittles demonstrated that the calculation of Wright's F_{st} statistic is biased towards smaller values due to a failure of certain core assumptions, such as equal population sizes among the subpopulations. They showed that, by relaxing those assumptions, F_{st} values may become larger. Nevertheless, they concluded that all human populations derive from a recent common ancestral group, that there is great genetic diversity within all human populations and that the geographic pattern of variation is complex and has no major discontinuities.[10] These points all that undermine the application of subspecies or race concepts to human populations.

In contrast, consider the subspecies differentiation of other mammalian species. Some large-bodied mammalian species show much higher values of population subdivision: white-tailed deer have a F_{st} of 0.60, the Grant's gazelle's F_{st} is 0.65 and North American grey wolves have a F_{st} of 0.75. Our closest relatives, chimpanzees and gorillas, also have much more subdivision between their populations than humans.[11] It would be legitimate to identify geographically based races in these particular mammalian species.

Various studies estimate that, during prehistoric times, our species spent most of its evolutionary time in a small region of northeastern Africa (70,000–100,000 out of 160,000–200,000 years). It was here that most of human genetic diversity evolved. As climates changed, successive groups of migrants left the region, and each migrating group by necessity contained only a part of the total accumulated genetic diversity. This loss of alleles during migration has been shown in other species as well.[12]

10 Jeffrey C. Long and Rick A. Kittles, 'Human genetic diversity and the non-existence of biological races', *Human Biology*, vol. 75, no. 4, August 2003, 449–71.
11 Henrik Kaessmann, Victor Wiebe and Svante Pääbo, 'Extensive nuclear DNA sequence diversity among chimpanzees', *Science*, vol. 286, 5 November 1999, 1159–62.
12 Sonya M. Clegg, Sandie M. Degnan, Jiro Kikkawa, Craig Moritz, Arnaud Estoup and Ian P. F. Owens, 'Genetic consequences of sequential founder events by an island-colonizing bird', *Proceedings of the National Academy of Sciences*, vol. 99, no. 12, June 2002, 8127–32.

Medical research is often conducted on a spurious racial basis

The absence of human races should be obvious, but the lack of scientific understanding of human population genetics among some researchers has led them to structure their studies as if conventional racial categories were biologically meaningful. The problems arising from such flawed data collection become obvious from close examination of the evidence that is used to support the 'human races' assumption. For example, some have argued that differences in the frequency of rare genetic diseases in socially defined races is positive proof that these groups can be reliably distinguished.[13] Others consistently err by assuming that biological differences that may exist between socially defined groups, such as disease incidence, are proof of an underlying genetic difference. Conversely, others make the mistake of believing that finding a genetic difference between socially defined groups automatically implies that such differences are responsible for whatever specific biological phenomenon they are studying.

Several studies have examined genetic variants that show large differences in frequency of hypertension between European and African-American populations, yet found no association between the alleles at candidate loci and the occurrence of hypertension.[14] While one can use non-coding portions of the genome to cluster human populations, this does not mean that these clusters coincide with socially defined racial groups, nor that these groups necessarily differ in genes that account for disease disparity between such socially defined groups.

For example, Hua Tang *et al.* utilized 326 microsatellite markers and found that they could cluster individuals of self-identified ancestry into groups that roughly corresponded with socially defined races. The details of such clustering are important, and indeed revelatory. Tang *et al.*'s study utilized the computer algorithm STRUCTURE. This piece of software allows users to define *in advance* how many clusters should exist at the end of the analysis. With the two-cluster option chosen at the start of the analysis, the software lumped self-identified individuals of African-American, Hispanic (Texas) and European ancestry together, the second cluster being made up of individuals who designated themselves as Chinese-American (Hawaii) and

13 Vincent Sarich and Frank Miele, *Race: The Reality of Human Differences* (Boulder, CO and Oxford: Westview 2004).
14 J. Barley, A. Blackwood, M. Miller, N. D. Markandu, N. D. Carter, S. Jeffery, F. P. Cappuccio, G. A. MacGregor and G. A. Sagnella, 'Angiotensin converting enzyme gene I/D polymorphism, blood pressure and the renin-angiotensin system in Caucasian and Afro-Caribbean peoples', *Journal of Human Hypertension*, vol. 10, no. 1, January 1996, 31–5; Hong-Guang Xie, C. Michael Stein, Richard B. Kim, James V. Gainer, Gbenga Sofowora, Victor Dishy, Nancy J. Brown, Robert E. Goree, Jonathan L. Haines and Alastair J. J. Wood, 'Human β2-adrenergic receptor polymorphisms: no association with essential hypertension in black and white Americans', *Clinical Pharmacology and Therapeutics*, vol. 67, no. 6, June 2000, 670–5.

Japanese-American (Stanford, CA). With the alternative three-cluster setting, the programme clustered African Americans separately from Hispanics and European Americans. With four clusters selected, a Hispanic cluster appeared in the output. It should be further noted that each of these three rather different clusterings included a few individuals who did not identify themselves as the majority of individuals in the inferred cluster. For example, cluster A, which was made up of 1,448 self-identified European Americans, also included three self-identified African Americans, one Hispanic and one person described as 'other'.[15]

A naive interpretation of these results supports the idea that medically significant genetic clustering exists within modern humans, and that these clusters reasonably coincide with self-identified race. But this interpretation is deeply flawed. The study was structured in a way that guaranteed that clustering would be found: the software was designed to cluster. Furthermore, the data were chosen so as to represent human populations that were either contemporaneously well separated or had geographically distinct recent origins. These groups, such as East Asians, Europeans and sub-Saharan Africans, are very far apart in the continuum of human genetic diversity. Furthermore, the roles of ancestry, genetic drift and geographically specific selection are conflated in such data. Non-coding portions of the genome may accumulate neutral mutations that are unrelated to how selection operates in coding portions, if these regions are far enough apart. For example, non-coding variation at eighty independent loci clustered Ashkenazi Jews very closely to Russians.[16] However, the genetically based disease distribution of the former is very different from the latter group.[17]

At present we do not have data that have been collected in a systematic way from the entire spectrum of human populations. For example, David Hinds et al. surveyed over two million single nucleotide polymorphisms in the human genome, but did *not* continuously sample human diversity. Instead, they examined DNA from individuals identified as African American, European American and Han Chinese.[18] Yet Africa, Europe and

15 Hua Tang, Tom Quertermous, Beatriz Rodriguez, Sharon L. R. Kardia, Xiaofeng Zhu, Andrew Brown, James S. Pankow, Michael A. Province, Steven C. Hunt, Eric Boerwinkle, Nicholas J. Schork and Neil J. Risch, 'Genetic structure, self-identified race/ethnicity, and confounding in case-control association studies', *American Journal of Human Genetics*, vol. 76, no. 2, February 2005, 268–75.

16 Sarah A. Tishkoff and Kenneth K. Kidd, 'Implications of biogeography of human populations for "race" and medicine', *Nature Genetics*, vol. 36, no. 11 (Supplement), November 2004, S21–S27.

17 Inbal Kedar-Barnes and Rozen Paul, 'The Jewish people: their ethnic history, genetic disorders and specific cancer susceptibility', *Familial Cancer*, vol. 3, nos 3–4, September 2004, 193–9.

18 David Hinds, Laura Stuve, Geoffrey Nilsen, Eran Halperin, Eleazar Eskin, Dennis Ballinger, Kelly Frazer and David Cox, 'Whole-genome patterns of common DNA variation in three human populations', *Science*, vol. 307, 18 February 2005, 1072–9.

Asia are large continents, while the ancestry of African Americans is primarily from a portion of the West Coast of Africa, Han Chinese represent only one ethnic Chinese group, and the ancestry of the European Americans in the study was not described. If one believes that biological races exist, and that Africa, Europe and Asia represent different biological races, then one might falsely believe that studies such as this one adequately characterize their genetic diversity. The authors of this paper did not claim that their findings revealed the detailed genetic structure of human populations. But many biomedical researchers act as if such systematically misleading samples adequately represent the spectrum of human diversity.

Many studies suggest that human genetic variation is continuous. Luigi Luca Cavalli-Sforza, Paolo Menozzi and Alberto Piazza illustrated this well in their use of maps of allele frequencies at multiple loci.[19] Their maps show continuous gradients in allele frequency from Africa to the Americas. Alan Templeton plots genetic distance versus geographic distance for 135 medically important loci. He found continuous change in genetic distance as a function of geographic distance between populations.[20] Clearly, the racial sampling of human genetic variation at widely separated points along its continuum greatly distorts the interpretation of geographic variation.

In another analysis of human population structure, Lynn Jorde and Stephen Wooding presented genetic data from individuals sampled from three geographically discontinuous regions.[21] They used 368 individuals of African, European and East Asian origin to study genetic variation within a 14,400 nucleotide sequence (14.4 kb) of the gene angiotensinogen (AGT). The alleles at this locus did not show statistically well-defined clustering. Another study that examined HLA alleles determined by DNA typing and sequencing in individuals from the Republic of Macedonia and Greece found that the Macedonians were more similar to an 'older' set of Mediterranean populations (Basques, North Africans, Italians, French, Cretans, Jews, Lebanese, Turks, Anatolians, Armenians and Iranians) and that the Greeks were closer to Ethiopians and sub-Saharan Africans (Oromo, Amhara, Fulani, Rimaibe and Mossi).[22] Thus, while individuals with shared

19 Luigi Luca Cavalli-Sforza, Paolo Menozzi and Alberto Piazza, *The History and Geography of Human Genes* (Princeton, NJ: Princeton University Press 1994). See also Alan R. Templeton, 'The genetic and evolutionary significance of human races', in Jefferson M. Fish (ed.), *Race and Intelligence: Separating Science from Myth* (Mahwah, NJ: Lawrence Erlbaum 2002); Frank B. Livingstone, 'On the non-existence of human races', *Current Anthropology*, vol. 3, no. 3, June 1962, 279–81.
20 Templeton, 'The genetic and evolutionary significance of human races'.
21 Lynn B. Jorde and Stephen P. Wooding, 'Genetic variation, classification, and race', *Nature Genetics*, vol. 36, no. 11 (Supplement), November 2004, S28–S33.
22 A. Arnaiz-Villena, K. Dimitroski, A. Pacho, J. Moscoso, E. Gómez-Casado, C. Silvera-Redondo, P. Varela, M. Blagoevska, V. Zdravkovska and J. Martínez-Laso, 'HLA genes in Macedonians and the sub-Saharan origin of the Greeks', *Tissue Antigens*, vol. 57, no. 2, February 2001, 118–27.

ancestry may be alike when it comes to correlations of large numbers of their genes, at any specific gene they may be different. In addition, the geographic proximity of populations doesn't always guarantee genetic relatedness at specific loci. These results argue against 'racial profiling' in medicine.

Patient populations are not genetically disjoint

The biological dubiousness of socially constructed races becomes most apparent when we discuss biomedical research. As mentioned above, human physical characteristics are not correlated with each other in ways that always reflect genetic relatedness. For this reason, we cannot necessarily infer that the genetic relatedness of individuals within populations means that they are certain to share the same disease phenotypes. Nor can we infer that the similarity of disease phenotypes among populations is proof that specific populations are more closely related to each other genetically than they are to other populations.

If we consider skin cancer incidence around the world, we observe a gradual increase as we move from the tropics towards the more northerly latitudes. We would be correct in surmising that this has something to do with skin colour. Northern European populations, which share specific alleles at melanin-producing loci but which also have cultural habits that encourage them to seek sunlight, should have similar rates among populations. Yet, when examined at multiple genetic loci, these European populations are closer genetically to indigenous Central American Indians than to sub-Saharan Africans. However, the sub-Saharan populations and the Central American Indians, while more genetically distant from each other, share lower skin cancer rates than Northern Europeans, both as a result of having more melanin in their skin and cultural habits that discourage exposure to sunlight. Finally, variation in skin colour is not necessarily correlated with variation for other physical traits. World skin colour shows approximately 88 per cent of its variation among regions, and only 12 per cent within regions, while fifty-seven craniometric measurements show 15 per cent of their variation among regions and 85 per cent of its variation within regions.[23]

But there is much more at stake than mere 'race identification' by practising physicians. A patient's social position and genetic ancestry may combine to produce predisposition to disease.[24] The United States was not founded by people who represented the complete spectrum of the world's genetic

23 John H. Relethford, 'Apportionment of global human genetic diversity based on craniometrics and skin color', *American Journal of Physical Anthropology*, vol. 118, no. 4, August 2002, 393–8.

24 Vicente Navarro, 'Race or class versus race and class: mortality differentials in the United States', *The Lancet*, vol. 336, no. 8725, 1990, 1238–40; Ichiro Kawachi, Norman Daniels and Dean E. Robinson, 'Health disparities by race and class: why both matter', *Health Affairs*, vol. 24, no. 2, March–April 2005, 343–52.

diversity. Initially, American society was composed of Northern Europeans, indigenous North Americans and Africans. Its first socially constructed races reflected who was there and their social position.

More recently, immigrants have arrived from regions such as the Middle East and Southeast Asia. In the face of such continuing immigration, the failure to study the full range of human genetic diversity will become more significant for the practice of medicine. Sampling large numbers of Europeans, followed by individuals from one region of China and even fewer individuals with ancestry from one portion of Africa, will produce findings that are of diminishing relevance to genetic predispositions to disease in the changing mixture of ancestries present in the United States. Furthermore, because of 'racial intermarriage', the rape of slaves and even the 'multiracial' ancestry of immigrants, one patient's self-proclaimed genetic ancestry may reflect well-defined origins in a specific portion of the world while this may not be true for other patients making the same claim of ancestry. For example, a study of self-reported race and genetic admixture showed that, while 93 per cent of those who self-identified as 'white' had a predominantly European genetic background, but only 4 per cent of those who self-identified as 'black' had a predominantly African genetic background.[25]

The study of 'nature *v.* nurture' in patients is complicated by socially constructed race

To what degree is health disparity between 'human races' the result of 'nature' and to what degree the result of 'nurture'? Almost every complex phenotype is produced by the interaction of genetic, environmental and chance events. Quantitative genetics is the tool that allows biologists to estimate the importance of each of these factors.

The case of the hypertension differential between American 'Blacks' and 'Whites' is one of the most reproducible findings for prospective racial medicine. The observation of elevated blood pressures in African Americans goes back to the early 1930s. By the 1960s similar observations had been made of Afro-Caribbeans. Many concluded that hypertension was a racial feature of 'the Negro', even as data were accumulating showing that no such elevated blood pressures could be found in Africans from West Africa and that there were European populations with similar rates of hypertension as African Americans. Various theories were proposed to explain black hypertension, including the salt retention hypothesis. Supposedly, hypertension was related to a historical absence of salt in West Africa, combined with the need for salt re-uptake in the survivors of the Middle Passage. By the early 1990s this theory had been widely adopted, with no published scientific data that

25 Moumita Sinha, Emma K. Larkin, Robert C. Elston and Susan Redline, 'Self-reported race and genetic admixture', *New England Journal of Medicine*, vol. 354, no. 4, January 2006, 421–2.

specifically supported its assertions. Subsequent analyses have dismantled the salt-hypertension hypothesis.[26]

If strong selection had been responsible for increased hypertension risk in Africans of the western hemisphere, we should see clear evidence of it in allele frequencies. At least 33 genetic systems and more than 63 genetic loci have been investigated for associations with increased risk of hypertension over the last six years. A recent search on MEDLINE showed 57 studies published between 1997 and 2003 that examined loci that might be associated with hypertension and racial variation. The results of these disparate studies can only be described as inconsistent, while their methodologies were often deficient. In only 7 out of the 57 studies were genetic variants consistently correlated with hypertension.[27]

A study of racial differences in drug action produced similarly inconsistent results. The study examined twenty-two drugs that had been claimed to show racial differentiation in medical outcome, including ACE inhibitors, vasodilators and beta-blockers. Despite the deliberate attempt to find racial genetic differences in drug effects, however, only one was found.[28]

Social dominance may create health disparities for socially constructed races

There is evidence that emotional stress can cause cellular damage.[29] A recent study demonstrated that greater susceptibility to cell deterioration arises among women caring for chronically ill children, relative to women caring for healthy children. Another recent study concludes that hypertension levels rise in African immigrants as they spend more time in white-dominated American or European societies.[30] Socially mediated stress can

26 Jay S. Kaufman and Susan A. Hall, 'The slavery hypertension hypothesis: dissemination and appeal of modern race theory', *Epidemiology*, vol. 14, no. 1, January 2003, 111–26.

27 Joseph L. Graves, Jr, *The Race Myth: Why We Pretend Race Exists in America* (New York: Dutton 2005), 126.

28 James F. Wilson, Michael E. Weale, Alice C. Smith, Fiona Gratrix, Benjamin Fletcher, Mark G. Thomas, Neil Bradman and David B. Goldstein, 'Population genetic structure of variable drug response', *Nature Genetics*, vol. 29, no. 3, November 2001, 265–9; Sarah K. Tate and David B. Goldstein, 'Will tomorrow's medicines work for everyone?', *Nature Genetics*, vol. 36, no. 11 (Supplement), November 2004, S34–S42.

29 Elissa S. Epel, Elizabeth H. Blackburn, Jue Lin, Firdaus S. Dhabhar, Nancy E. Adler, Jason D. Morrow and Richard M. Cawthon, 'Accelerated telomere shortening in response to life stress', *Proceedings of the National Academy of Sciences*, vol. 101, no. 49, December 2004, 17312–15.

30 Jen'nan Ghazal Read, Michael O. Emerson and Alvin Tarlov, 'Implications of black immigrant health for U.S. racial disparities in health', *Journal of Immigrant Health*, vol. 7, no. 3, July 2005, 205-12; Jen'nan Ghazal Read and Michael O. Emerson, 'Racial context of origin, black immigration, and the U.S. black/white health disparity', *Social Forces*, vol. 84, no. 1, September 2005, 183–201.

cause illness, and such stress may be partly dependent on socially ascribed racial status. But these are only initial findings. We need to know more; medical research should address the impact of socially assigned race on health.

Another study has estimated how much the United States has to gain by eliminating health disparities among socially designated races. It compared the number of lives saved by advances in medical technology from 1991 to 2000 with the number of lives that could have been 'saved' by equalizing 'black' and 'white' mortality rates over the same period. The difference was 886,202 more lives spared without health disparity.[31] At a minimum, this finding suggests that there is a need for considerable redirection of biomedical research and public health resources towards the role of perceived race in health outcomes. This should not be interpreted as opposition to basic research on human genetics. However, if we are going to address health disparity with limited funds to achieve our ends, we need to take account of what is going to improve health the most.

Medicine should take both social environment and population genetics into account, not spurious 'human races' that inappropriately conflate the two

Human genetic variation is real. Individuals with ancestry in particular geographic regions are more likely to share genes with other individuals from the same region. But the overall amount of measured genetic differentiation between human populations is meagre. In particular, living as a 'black person' or a 'white person' in the United States may lead to substantially different health outcomes, regardless of underlying genetic differences. Modern human population genetic research demonstrates that apportioning individuals into racial groups, particularly those groupings defined by our historical conceptions of 'race', is a dubious enterprise. Dangerous consequences may follow from the implementation of racial medicine in clinical practice. In addition to fostering social inequality by underscoring racial classification, racial medicine might kill people by neglecting the substantial genetic variation within, and genetic overlap between, human populations.

31 Steven H. Woolf, Robert E. Johnson, George E. Fryer, Jr, George Rust and David Satcher, 'The health impact of resolving racial disparities: an analysis of US mortality data', *American Journal of Public Health*, vol. 94, no. 12, December 2004, 2078–81.

Joseph L. Graves, Jr is Dean of University Studies and Professor of Biological Sciences at North Carolina Agricultural and Technical State University, Greensboro. He is a fellow of the American Association for the Advancement of Science.

Michael R. Rose is Director of the University of California Network for Experimental Research on Evolution, and Professor of Biological Sciences at the University of California, Irvine.

Index

academic classifications; heritable disease 92
addiction; alcoholism 38
African American: demographic groups 98;
    DNA 2; habits 116; intelligence 101; mistrust
    98–9; women 165
Alcabes, P. x
alcohol; Jews 32–49, 40–9
alcoholism: addiction 38; causes 35–6; gene for
    resistance to 36–8; genes 35–40; Jews 35
allele; presence 24–6
Allport, G. 92–3
American Anthropological Association 34–5
Amudha, K. 55
ancestral condition 83
ancestry: DNA 11; genetics 11; genomic 14, 15;
    medical relevance 9; race 162; Sephardic 89
Ashkenazic Jews 36–7
Asians; lung cancer 127
AstraZeneca 127
Azouley, K.G. x

Bales, R. 48–9
Barrett, A. 57–8
Bascombe, D. 134
behaviour; myths 115–16
Bell Curve: Intelligence and Class Structure in
    American Life (Hernstein and Murray) 169
bias; aesthetic and political 59
BiDil 2, 124, 125–7; clinical trial 125–6; ethnic
    drug 61; NitroMed 9; race specific 127;
    research data 15
bio-piracy 18
biobanks 143–7; race-marking 152–4; racial 137–54
biocolonialism 18
biocomputing 140
biological difference theory 168
biological encoding; shortcomings 96
biological fiction; social fact 59–62
biological races 178–9
biologization: difference 50–76; identity 72; race 61
biology: definition 11–13; limits 95–9; race 128–9
biomedical research; race 150–2
biotechnology 21; forensic science 123–36
blood ties; rabbinic law 90
bone marrow donors; shortage 64
Bone Marrow Project; MatchMaker 64
Book of Icelanders; database 144
Bordenave, K. 83
breast cancer: genomics 161; mortality rates for
    black women 168; race 155–74; racialized
    discourse 163–73; research 155–74, 163–73;
    research racialism 173; statistical anomaly 156;
    susceptibility 167
Bruns, P.J. 41–2, 43–4
Bushman, S. 22, 23

Caucasian; origin 71
Cavalli-Sforza, L.L. 16, 182
cellular damage; emotional stress 195–6

Census; federal document 65
characteristics: cultural 79; heritable 79
chatel slavery 177
chip technology 128
cholera; disease 114
Choy, A.M. 55
chromosomes; Y markers 81
classification; human 93
clinical drug trials; race 8–10
clinical research; mistrust 98–9
Clinton, President W. 141–2
CODIS; database 133
Cohen gene 73
Collins, F. 31, 142
colour-blind: analysis 160, 162; research 147–50
community: disability 107–8; faith 92
cranial capacity; intelligence measure 59
Creutzfeldt-Jakob Disease (CJD): genetic links
    79–94; heritable 89; legend 87
criminality; mark 136
crypto-Jewish descent 81
crypto-Jewish lineage 88
CSI; TV series 62–4
culture: ethnicity 53–9; race 53–9

Darwinian theory 117
database; Book of Icelanders 144
Davenport, C. 176
deCode Genetics 144
defective genes; eugenics 103
definition; biology 11–13
demographic groups; African Americans 98
determinism; genetic 119
diasporic patterns 89
difference: biologicalization 50–76; disease 119;
    making sense of 50–3
Dinoire, I.; face transplant viii
disability: community 107–8; discrimination 96–7;
    experiences 107–8; genetic science 102; genetic
    testing 103; genomics 107–8; inferiority 96;
    mistrust 99; movement 107; notions 105; race 96,
    96–7, 97–100; statistics 97; studies 102; voices of
    the people 107–8
disabled people 95–7
discrimination; disability 96–7
disease: behavioural causes 121; cholera 114;
    differences 119; heritable 79, 91, 92, 93; Jewish
    86–91; Juddism 90; metaphor 119; reducing 113;
    religious descent 91–2; resistance 38–9; risk 112,
    113; Sephardi 88; susceptibility 117–18;
    tuberculosis (TB) 114–15; yellow fever 115
disorders; Mendalian 158
disparity: environmental risk factors 156;
    health 186
diversity; approach 100
DNA 18, 22; African Americans 2; ancestry 11;
    databanks 132–5; evidence 23; forensic database
    134; Polymorphism Discovery Resource (PDR)
    147; population-wide databases 135–6;

post-conviction cases 123; racial labeling 152; repositories 139, 140; samples storage 131; sequencing issues 74; United Kingdom (UK) 133–4
Dobzhansky, T. 6
drug action; study 185
Du Bois, W.E.B. 137
Duster, T. *x* 7, 14

emotional stress; cellular damage 195–6
Enlightenment 40
environmental risk factors; disparity 156
epidemics: African American 115; race 113–16; resistance to 115; social conditions 114
epidemiologist's model; genticist model 120
epidemiology: behavioural 112–13; evolution 116–19; race 110–21; risk 110–11; use and origins 111–12
Esther, Persian Jews 41
ethnic classification 7
ethnic drug; BiDil 61
ethnicity: culture 53–9; definition 33; genetic basis 33; race 5–7, 53–9, 124
eugenics: African American institutions 106; defective genes 103; genetics 101–4; human pedigree 105; institutionalized 101; interventionist projects 104; movement 99, 100–1
euthanasia; Nazi 118
Evett, I. 131; and Lowe, A. 129
evolution: epidemiology 116–19; geographical changes 26; misreading 110
evolutionary theory 116
exploitation 19–21

face transplant; Dinoire, I. *viii*
faith community; genetic labeling 92
Fields, B. 68
Figgs, L. 173–4
fingerprints; collection of 135
Fishberg, M. 48
FOAFtale (Friend-of-a-Friend): legends 84–6, 87; modern Spanish-American 90
folk; taxonomy 77–94, 91–4
folk logic; elements 87
folklore analysis 85–6
Food and Drug Administration (FDA) 9; guidelines 151; role 69
forensic science: biotechnology 123–36; segue 129–31
founder mutations: detections 166; frequency 164
Fredrickson, G. 96
freedom; bondage 67
Friedländer, D. 43–4

Gannett, L.; populational thinking 153
Gates, H.L. *vii-viii*
genes: alcoholism 35–40; candidate 128; definitions 1
genetic data; mapping 105
genetic deviance; identification 100
genetic drift; tracing 100
genetic labelling; faith community 92
genetic links; Creutzfeldt-Jakob Disease (CJD) 79–94
genetic particularity 139–40

genetic project: Iceland 146; Korea 146
genetic science; disability 102
genetic signature 72; language 75
genetic testing; disability 103
genetic trail 23, 27
genetic variation 6; mapping 32
geneticists; population 16–17
genetics: ancestry 11; critique 106; determinism 119; drifts 16–17; eugenics 101–4; interventions 106–7; knowledge 107; national merging 145–6; population 6, 10–11, 186; quantitative 184–5; race 15, 140–3; screening 130; surveillance 134
Genographic Project 21
genome research 104
genome variation; human 17
genomic information 11, 30; migration 23; misuse 4–6
genomic medicine: goal 20; migration 31; practice 30; race 10–12
Genomic Research of the African Diaspora (GRAD) 97
genomic variation 8, 18; race 4–8
genomics 1–31; ancestry 14, 15; breast cancer 161; disability 107–8; population 14, 21, 25; populations 31; racism 3; research 3, 9–11, 21–8
genticist model; epidemiologist's model 120
geographical changes; evolution 26
Germany; Nazi 124
Gilroy, P. 76
Giuliani, R. 134
globalization; human mixture 29
Goodman, R.M. 89
Gould, S.J. 106
Graham, S. 63
Graves, J.L.; and Rose, M.R. *x*
Gutiérrez, R. 80

Hall, S. 3
HapMap project 158, 159
Happe, K.E. *x*
Haraway, D. 161
Harrell, J. 61–2
health: disparities 124; disparity 186; ethnicity-specific 33
health-based comparisons 99
hereditarily susceptible 121
hereditary trait; laziness 176
heritable characteristics 79
heritable disease 79, 91; academic classifications 92; categorizing differences 93; marker 84; markers 81, 82–4
heterosexual unions; perceptions 59–60
heterosexual relations 67
Hinds, D. 181
Hispanic; racial classification 63
history; racial theory 67
Howard University; Washington 152–4
human classification 93
human genome 91–3; mapping 123; patterns within 91; prejudice 77–94; research 99–101; sequencing 123
Human Genome Diversity Project (HGDP) 17–19, 20
Human Genome Project (HGP) 17, 101, 106, 141; media 101; rationale behind 123

human genomics; racial interpretations 121
human groups; conceptual organizing 173
human mixture; globalization 29
human pedigree: charts 104–5; eugenics 105;
    hereditary 104–7
human valuation 78
human variation: categories 78–80; folk categories
    78–80
Hume, D. 45
hypertension differential; research 184
hypo descent; on-drop rule 177

Iceland; genetic project 146
identification: genetic deviance 100; race 177–8
identity; biologization 72
indigenous groups 26–8
Indigenous Peoples Council on Biocolonialism
    (IPCB) 19
indigenous world-view 23
industrial revolution 113–14
inequities; social and economic 29
inferiority: built-in 96; disability 96; racial 96, 115
intelligence; African American 101
intelligence measure; cranial capacity 59
internet 122–4
intervention: genetics 106–7; legislative 67
interventionist projects; eugenics 104
IPCB 24
Iressa 124, 127–8

Jacobs, L. 88–90
Jews: alcohol 32–49, 40–9; alcoholism 35; Poland 47
Jorde, L.; and Wooding, S. 182
Juddism; disease 90

Kant, I. 46–7, 49
Keller, E.F. 140, 161
Kelly, P.J. 133
Kerr, N. 48
Kidd, K.K. 4
Kittles, R. 179
Klag, M. 127
knowledge; genetics 107
Korea; genetic project 146
Krieger, N. 156, 170

Latino; racial classification 63
Latour, B. 150
Lavater, J.C.; Mendelssohn, M. 41
Lee, S. S-J. x
legend: constructing 84–6; Creutzfeldt-Jakob
    Disease (CJD) 87; crypto-Jews 85; FAOFtale 84–6,
    87; Niemann-Pick 86–8; urban 84
Lemba 72
Leroi, A. 159, 177
Lessing, G.E. 41
Lewontin, R. 8; and Montagu, A. 158
Libyan Jews 86–90
Lindee, S.; and Nelkin, D. ix
lineage; crypto-Jewish 88
Linneaus, C. 74
Loewnthal, R. 83
Long, J. 179
Lowe, A.; and Evett, I. 129
lung cancer; Asians 127

Man's Most Dangerous, Myth (Montagu) 51
mantra; sameness 153
mapping: genetic variation 32;
    human genome 123
marker: ethnic 83; heritable disease 81, 82–4;
    Sephardi 90, 91
Marks, J. 159
MatchMaker; Bone Marrow Project 64
matrilineal descent 87–8
MAVIN Foundation 64
media; Human Genome Project (GJP) 101
medical research: racial basis 180–3;
    racial profiling 176
medicalization; race 71
medication: prescribing 32; race 32
medicine; racial 176–86
Medicine and the German Jews (Efron) 35–6
Mendalian; disorders 158
Mendelssohn, M.; Lavater, J.C. 41
metaphor; disease 119
miasma theory 114
migration: genomic information 23; genomic
    medicine 31; human 16; human routes 21–8;
    human 18
mistrust: African American 98–9;
    disability 99
Mitchell, D.T.; and Snyder, S.L. x
mixed race; racial classification 63
molecular level; politics 95–108
molecular reinscription; race 123
Montagu, A. 51, 54–5, 178; and Lewontin, R. 158
movement: disability 107; eugenics 99, 100–1
multiracial category; advocates 65
myth: behaviour 115–16; race 51; racism 11;
    science 27

narrative 84
National Human Genome Centre (NHGC) 1–2, 4
natural selection; principle 117
nature; nurture 184–5
Nature Biotechnology 154
Nazis: euthanasia 118; Germany 124
Nazis' Final Solution 118
Negro; status 66
Nelkin, D.; and Lindee, S. ix
Neulander, J.S. x
New Mexican crypto Jews 80–4
Niemann-Pick; legend 86–8
NitroMed 61, 126; BiDil 9
nurture; nature 184–5

offenders; SNP profiling 136
Omi, M.; and Winant, H. 157
on-drop rule; hypo descent 177
Operation Pipleline 128–9
over-generalization; genetic 80

patient; populations 183–4
pharmaceuticals; testing 35
pigmentocracy 84–90
Poland; Jews 47
polarization; black-white 110
political correctness 12–13
politicization; sex 60
politics; molecular level 95–108

Polymorphism Discovery Resource (PDR): DNA 147; resource samples 147–8
popularization; race 62–5
population: geneticists 16–17; genetics 6, 10–11, 186; genomics 14, 21, 25, 31; patient 183–4
populational thinking; Gannett, L. 153
prejudice: human genome 77–94; taxonomy 91–4
preservation; cultural 29
Project Race 63–4
psychological comparison; race 70
Purim 42, 43–4, 45

rabbinic law 88; blood ties 90
race 34, 50–76; academic friction 60; ancestry 162; biological basis 30–1; biological category 125; biologization 61; biology 128–9; biomedical research 150–2; breast cancer 155–74; categories 117; clinical drug trials 8, 8–10; culture 53–9; disability 96, 96–7, 97–100; epidemics 113–16; epidemiology 111–21; ethnicity 5–7, 53–9, 124; genetics 15, 140–3; genomic medicine 10–12; genomic variation 4–8; grammar 66–8; identification 177–8; inferiority 96; letting go 75–6; meaning 162–3; meaning and origin 34; medicalization 71; medication 32; metaphor 119–21; molecular reinscription 123; myth 51; navigating 125–31; popularization 62–5; as proxy 28–31; psychological comparison 70; pure 142; rhetorical significance 157–63; scientific concept 130; scientific study 5; self-identified 12; social construction 53; social-political construct 65; unlearning 68–72
race-making 138; biobanks 152–4
racial classification 7; criteria 60; Hispanic/Latino 63; history 2; immutable 61; mixed race 63
racial discrimination 69
racial genome; eugenics 95–108
racial interpretations; human genomics 121
racial labeling; DNA 152
racial profiling: medical research 176; research 176
racial theory; history 67
racialized discourse; breast cancer 163–73
racialized society; living in 61
racial groups; indentifying 98
racing 66
racism 18; biological 97; genomics 3; history 7–8, 31; medical impact 14; myths 11; problem of 6; science 1; scientific 29–31; social consequences 13–14
religious descent; disease 91–2
religious labels 78
repositories; DNA 139, 140
research: breast cancer 155–74, 163–73; colour-blind 147–50; genomics 3, 9–11, 21–8; human genome 99–101; hypertension differential 184; racial profiling 176; self reporting 37
residual confounding; problem of 169
resource samples; Polymorphism Discovery Resource (PDR) 147–8
Risch, N. 10–13, 150–1, 165
risk 110–12; behavioural disease 112; disease 112, 113; epidemiology 110–11
Romtimi, C. 33
Rose, M.R.; and Graves, J.L. *x*
Ross, R. 117

Safir, H.; New York Police Chief 134
sameness; mantra 153
Samuelson, J. 48
Schudt, J.J. 42
Schwartz, R.; and Wood, A. 176
science: local 99–101; myth 27; racism 1; story 24; universal 99–101
scientific concept; race 130
scientific study; race 5
scientific knowledge; production 112
screening; genetics 130
seed-and-soil metaphor 118
Sephardi: ancestry 89; disease 88; marker 90, 91
sex; politicization 60
shibboleth 55
shortcomings; biologically encoded 96
sickle-cell anemia 167
single nucleotide polymorphisms (SNPs) 138
skin cancer; incidence 183
slavery 66–7
Snyder, S.L.; and Mitchell, D.T. *x*
social conditions; epidemics 114
social construction 53; race 53
social dominance; health role 185
social fact; biological fiction 59–62
social pressures 3
Social Security (USA) 132
social stratification; disease rates 120
social-political construct; race 65
Spanish Jews 78–84
status; Negro 66
story; science 24
studies; disability 102
susceptibility; disease 117–18
Sutton, W. 7, 83
Systema Naturae (Linneaus) 177

Tang, H. 162; socially defined races 180
taxonomy: folk 77–94, 91–4; prejudice 91–4
testing; pharmaceuticals 35
Thompson, S. 85
Tishkoff, S.A. 4
Transeau, E. 47
tuberculosis (TB); disease 114–15
Tuskegee experiment 176
TV series; *CSI* 62–4

unique mutations; reference to 166
United Kingdom (UK); DNA 133–4
United States of America (USA); health data 111
US Census 63

Venter, C. 142
von Humboldt, W. 42
von Knigge, A.F. 45–6

Wailoo, K. 139
Wald, P. *x*
Washington; Howard University 152–4
white privilege 69
Williams, P. 51–2
Winant, H.; and Omi, M. 157
Wirght, S. 178
women; African American 165
Women's Christian Temperance Union 40

Wong, L.P. 55
Wood, A.; and Schwartz, R. 176
Wooding, S.; and Jorde, L. 182
World Wide Web 123
Wyatt, S. 61

yellow fever; disease 115
Young, R. 68

Zack, N. 143
Zimmerman, E. 176